NEUROSCIENCE RESEARCH PROGRESS

PREFRONTAL CORTEX

DEVELOPMENTAL DIFFERENCES, EXECUTIVE AND COGNITIVE FUNCTIONS AND ROLE IN NEUROLOGICAL DISORDERS

NEUROSCIENCE RESEARCH PROGRESS

Additional books in this series can be found on Nova's website under the Series tab.

Additional e-books in this series can be found on Nova's website under the e-book tab.

NEUROSCIENCE RESEARCH PROGRESS

PREFRONTAL CORTEX

DEVELOPMENTAL DIFFERENCES, EXECUTIVE AND COGNITIVE FUNCTIONS AND ROLE IN NEUROLOGICAL DISORDERS

ROBERT O. COLLINS
AND
JOHN L. ADAMS
EDITORS

NOVA BIOMEDICAL

New York

For permission to use material from this book please contact us:
Telephone 631-231-7269; Fax 631-231-8175
Web Site: http://www.novapublishers.com

Additional color graphics may be available in the e-book version of this book.

Library of Congress Cataloging-in-Publication Data

ISBN: 978-1-62618-663-7

Library of Congress Control Number: 2013935916

Published by Nova Science Publishers, Inc. † New York

CONTENTS

Preface

The prefrontal cortex (PFC) is the anterior part of the frontal lobes of the brain, lying in front of the motor and premotor areas and has been implicated in planning complex cognitive behavior, personality expression, decision making and moderating social behavior. In this book, the authors discuss the developmental differences, executive and cognitive functions and role in neurological disorders relating to the functioning of the prefrontal cortex. Topics include developmental long-chain omega-3 fatty acid deficiency and prefrontal cortex pathology in psychiatric disorders; addiction and the prefrontal cortex; cognitive functioning and prefrontal cortex damage in children and adolescents; prefrontal cortex dysfunction and neurocognitive deficits in schizophrenia; and the developmental relationship between executive function and the prefrontal cortex in young children.

Chapter 1 - Major psychiatric disorders including unipolar and bipolar depression, schizophrenia, and attention deficit hyperactivity disorder share cognitive impairments associated with deficits prefrontal cortex (PFC) structure and function. These disorders commonly initially emerge during adolescence, a period associated with rapid and dynamic changes in PFC structural maturation. Increasing evidence also suggests that each of these psychiatric disorders are associated with a deficiency in long-chain omega-3 (LC*n*-3) fatty acids, including eicosapentaenoic acid (EPA, 20:5*n*-3) and docosahexaenoic acid (DHA, 22:6*n*-3), which are evident proximal to illness onset. Preclinical studies have demonstrated LC*n*-3 fatty acids and their bioactive lipid metabolites have central neurotrophic, ant-inflammatory, and neuroprotective properties, and that reducing cortical DHA accrual during perinatal development leads to enduring deficits in PFC biochemistry and function. Preliminary human neuroimaging studies also suggest that LC*n*-3 fatty acid status is positively associated with cortical structural and functional integrity. Together, this body of translational evidence supports the proposition that low LC*n*-3 fatty acid status during active periods of PFC maturation may represent a modifiable pathogenic mechanism leading to deficits in PFC structure and function associated with psychopathology.

Chapter 2 - Addiction is usually defined as the continued use of substances or activities despite their negative consequences. Different models have been proposed to explain why people start using drugs and why they still continue using even when they experience physical, psychological and/or social problems. In this context, prefrontal cortex (PFC), which has been involved in complex cognitive functions such as abstract thinking, planning, inhibitory control or decision-making, has gained much of the attention when explaining addiction due to its implication in different aspects related to addictives behaviours. In this chapter, the authors will focus on the PFC and its involvement in the addictives processes, paying particular attention to the somatic marker hypothesis. According to this model, substance abusers as well as patients with ventromedial prefrontal cortex (VMPC) lesions, show altered decision-making, characterized by a tendency to choose the immediate reward and by not taking into account long-term consequences of their behaviour. Growing scientific evidence indicates that core aspects of addiction may be explained in terms of an abnormal decision-making. The aim of this chapter is to review the previous literature regarding the role of the PFC in this process and, therefore, in the addictive behaviour. After describing the anatomy and functions of the PFC, different models and definitions of addiction will be discussed. Then, the authors will focus on the somatic marker model, which establishes that the altered decision-making in addiction is a consequence of an abnormal functioning of a distributed neural network critical for the processing of emotional information involving several regions of the PFC and limbic system. Accordingly, an examination of the scientific evidences that support the role of PFC in addiction will be conducted. Finally, the authors will discuss the implications for addiction treatment and prevention.

Chapter 3 - Several lines of evidence suggest that pathological alterations in specific neuronal circuits within the prefrontal cortex (PFC), including those inter-connecting the PFC and the mesial temporal lobe, may result in impaired neurocognitive functioning in schizophrenia (SZ) patients. These pathological alterations are thought to arise via disturbances in early neurodevelopmental and neural migratory processes, and ultimately degrade the efficiency of neural networks and thereby impair cognition. Recent reports have identified different neural substrates that are impacted by these aberrant neurodevelopmental processes, and these substrates are being explored as potential targets for pro-cognitive pharmacologic interventions in SZ. A number of cognitive, behavioral and pharmacological interventions modestly enhance neurocognitive function to some degree in SZ patients. Here, the authors consider opportunities for optimizing PFC performance, to enable residual healthy circuitry to maximize benefits from these interventions, and thereby improve neurocognition in SZ.

Chapter 4 - Traumatic brain injury (TBI) is a major problem of public health around the world since it is the first cause of death among children and adolescents in most of the developed countries. TBI is a neurological disorder that results in temporary or permanent changes in motor, cognitive and behavioral areas. TBI is one of the most common kinds of brain injuries in childhood/adolescence, a period in which the prefrontal cortex is in a developing process. The aim of this chapter is to review neuropsychological consequences of TBI in prefrontal cortex during childhood/adolescence, as well as the valid strategies to be adopted that might contribute to a shorter recovery time of the young people in development. The TBI in the prefrontal cortex does not involve motor or sensorial deficits. However, it can cause functional, social and academic impairments. More than a half of these children/adolescents develop a psychiatric disorder with disinhibiting symptoms and inappropriate behavior. Motivational, emotional, attention, perceptive and cognitive functions are mediated by the connections between the prefrontal cortex and the motor areas, the limbic system, the reticular system and the posterior association cortex. Generally, patients with TBI will present cognitive deficits associated with executive functions, decision making, problem solving skills, judgment and impulse control. The consequences of brain injury in childhood/adolescence depend on a variety of factors, such as: the type of brain injury, intensity of the damage, extension, localization, environmental factors, age in which the TBI occurs, premorbid intelligence/cognitive reserve, and stage of cognitive development. For example, dorsolateral lesions have been associated with perseverative behavior, lack of initiative, deficit in ability to sustain and shift attention between stimuli or concepts, problem solving and working memory ("cold" executive functions). It is commonly confused with unmotivated behavior. On the other hand, ventromedial injuries have been associated with conducts based on emotional and social variables, such as inability to respond appropriately to social cues, failure to obey conventional social rules, inhibitory deficits, impulsivity and impaired decision making ("hot" executive functions).

Chapter 5 - Executive function refers to the ability to plan and execute task-relevant actions and to inhibit irrelevant actions for the attainment of a specific goal. Extensive adult neuroimaging research has revealed that the lateral prefrontal cortex plays an important role in executive function. Recently, developmental studies have shown behavioral evidence that executive function changes significantly during preschool years. It has been proposed that the maturation of the prefrontal cortex plays an essential role in the development of executive function. However, there is little evidence to support this proposal. The authors have used near-infrared spectroscopy to examine the relationship between the development of executive function and the lateral prefrontal cortex. In this article, the authors show how the development of executive function is related to the lateral prefrontal cortex from the perspective of developmental cognitive neuroscience. Four studies examined the relationship between executive function and the prefrontal cortex in young children. First, the authors showed that prefrontal activation correlated with performance on executive function tasks in young children with the Dimensional Change Card Sort (DCCS). Second, the authors investigated the longitudinal relationship between the prefrontal cortex and executive function in young children and found that children showed better behavioral performance and significantly stronger inferior prefrontal activation at 4 years of age than they did at 3 years of age. Moreover, the authors demonstrated individual differences in the development of prefrontal activation. Third, the authors revealed that the prefrontal cortex was activated differently depending on task demands. Fourth, the authors compared the behavioral and neural responses in typically developing children to children with autism and found that children with autism showed decreased behavioral performances and less activation in the prefrontal area during the DCCS task than typically developing children did. Taken together, these results suggested that the development of executive function might be strongly related to the prefrontal cortex in preschool-aged children. These results contribute to the author's general understanding of the pathway of cognitive development during early childhood and may lead to the support of and interventions for children with developmental disorders.

In: Prefrontal Cortex
Editors: R. O. Collins and J. L. Adams
ISBN 978-1-62618-663-7

Chapter 1

Developmental Long-Chain Omega-3 Fatty Acid Deficiency and Prefrontal Cortex Pathology in Psychiatric Disorders

Robert K. McNamara*

Department of Psychiatry and Behavioral Neuroscience, University of Cincinnati College of Medicine, Cincinnati, OH, US

Abstract

Major psychiatric disorders including unipolar and bipolar depression, schizophrenia, and attention deficit hyperactivity disorder share cognitive impairments associated with deficits prefrontal cortex (PFC) structure and function. These disorders commonly initially emerge during adolescence, a period associated with rapid and dynamic changes in PFC structural maturation. Increasing evidence also suggests that each of these psychiatric disorders are associated with a deficiency in long-chain omega-3 (LC*n*-3) fatty acids, including eicosapentaenoic acid (EPA, 20:5*n*-3) and docosahexaenoic acid (DHA, 22:6*n*-3), which are evident proximal to illness onset. Preclinical studies have demonstrated

* Corresponding author: Robert K. McNamara, Ph.D., Department of Psychiatry and Behavioral Neuroscience, University of Cincinnati College of Medicine, 260 Stetson Street, Cincinnati, OH 45219-0516. PH: 513-558-5601; FAX: 513-558-4805; E-mail: robert.mcnamara@uc.edu.

LC*n*-3 fatty acids and their bioactive lipid metabolites have central neurotrophic, ant-inflammatory, and neuroprotective properties, and that reducing cortical DHA accrual during perinatal development leads to enduring deficits in PFC biochemistry and function. Preliminary human neuroimaging studies also suggest that LC*n*-3 fatty acid status is positively associated with cortical structural and functional integrity. Together, this body of translational evidence supports the proposition that low LC*n*-3 fatty acid status during active periods of PFC maturation may represent a modifiable pathogenic mechanism leading to deficits in PFC structure and function associated with psychopathology.

INTRODUCTION

Major psychiatric disorders including major depressive disorder (MDD), bipolar disorder, schizophrenia, and attention deficit hyperactivity disorder (ADHD), are prominent causes of premature disability and mortality. In the United States (U.S.), severe forms of MDD currently affect between 2-7%, and up to 16-20% suffer from milder forms of the illness, and life-time prevalence estimates for bipolar disorder are 1.0% for bipolar-I, 1.1% for bipolar-II, and 2.4% for subthreshold bipolar disorder (4.4% total)(Kessler et al., 2007). In the U.S., ADHD is one of the most common childhood psychiatric disorders with prevalence rates ranging from 5-16% (http://www.cdc.gov/ncbddd/adhd/prevalence.html), and schizophrenia has a life-time prevalence rate of approximately 1.0% (McGuffin et al., 2004). These psychiatric disorders are chronic and typically recurring illnesses associated with significant psychosocial morbidity, and mood and psychotic disorders are associated with excess premature mortality attributable primarily to suicide and cardiovascular-related diseases (Angst et al., 2002; Brown et al., 1997; Osby et al., 2001). These disorders also have a significant economic impact due in part to excess health care utilization (Greenburg et al., 2003; Kleinman et al., 2003; Meyers et al., 2010; Wu et al., 2005). Psychiatric symptoms typically require long-term treatment with pharmacological agents and symptomatic relapse following medication discontinuation is common (Ayuso-Gutierrez & del Rio Vega, 1997; Cavanagh et al., 2004; Geddes et al., 2003). Therefore, developing a better understanding of the risk and resilience mechanisms associated with the initial development of psychopathology represents an urgent public health need.

The pathogenic mechanisms underlying major psychiatric disorders are viewed as polygenic and multifactorial. Indeed, subtotal heritability estimates and monozygotic twin discordance rates indicate that both genetic and environmental factors confer vulnerability and offspring of first degree relatives with mood or psychotic disorders have an elevated risk of developing psychiatric disorders (Ehringer et al., 2006; Sullivan et al., 2000; Tsuang et al., 2000). An important clue into the pathoetiology of psychiatric disorders may come from when they initially emerge during the lifespan. Specifically, the initial onset of major mood and psychotic disorders frequently occur during adolescence or early adulthood (Burke et al., 1991; Kessler et al., 2005; Perlis et al., 2009), a developmental period associated with rapid and dynamic changes in prefrontal cortex (PFC) structural maturation in typically developing youth (Geidd et al., 2009). Specifically, the period between childhood and early adolescence (7-12 years) is associated with the rapid expansion of gray matter density in the PFC, and the period between adolescence (13-18 years) and young adulthood (≥18 years) is associated with a progressive loss of cortical gray matter density and reciprocal increases in white matter density in fronto-temporal fiber tracts (Geidd et al., 2009). Consistent with a neurodevelopmental etiology, converging evidence from cross-sectional and longitudinal structural magnetic resonance imaging (MRI) studies have found that psychiatric disorders including MDD (Bora et al., 2012; Drevets, 2000; Sacher et al., 2012), bipolar disorder (Schneider et al., 2012; Strakowski et al., 2012), schizophrenia (De Peri et al., 2012; Vita et al., 2013), and ADHD (Castellanos et al., 2002; Helpern et al., 2011; Shaw & Rabin, 2009), are associated with deficits in PFC functional integrity and associated abnormalities in connectivity with limbic and striatal structures. Therefore, the initial onset of major psychiatric disorders coincides with active and dynamic changes in PFC structural maturation, and perturbations in these maturational processes may contribute to the emergence of psychopathology.

While the risk and resilience mechanisms associated with abnormal PFC development in psychiatric disorders remain poorly understood, a substantial body of evidence has emerged over the last twenty years which suggest that psychiatric disorders including MDD, bipolar disorder, schizophrenia, and ADHD, are associated with deficits in long-chain omega-3 (LC*n*-3) fatty acids compared with healthy controls. Moreover, emerging evidence from preclinical studies and preliminary human MRI studies suggest that LC*n*-3 fatty acid deficiency during perinatal development impacts PFC structural and functional integrity. The objective of this chapter is to critically evaluate translational evidence implicating LC*n*-3 fatty acids in PFC development and explore potential relevance to the PFC abnormalities observed in psychiatric patients.

LC*n*-3 Fatty Acid Deficiency and Psychiatric Disorders

As background, mammals require a dietary source of *n*-3 fatty acids to procure and maintain adequate concentrations of LC*n*-3 fatty acids in peripheral and central tissues. Principal dietary sources of the vegetable short-chain *n*-3 fatty acid precursor α-linolenic acid (ALA, 18:3*n*-3) include flaxseed, linseed, canola, soy, and perilla oils. The biosynthesis of LC*n*-3 fatty acids, including eicosapentaenoic acid (EPA, 20:5*n*-3) and docosahexaenoic acid (DHA, 22:6*n*-3), from ALA requires a series of microsomal reactions mediated by desaturase and elongase enzymes/genes. The rate-limiting enzymes regulating LC*n*-3 fatty acid biosynthesis include delta-6 desaturase (*Δ*6-desaturase, *FADS2*) and delta-5 desaturase (*Δ*5-desaturase, *FADS1*), and emerging evidence from human genotyping studies suggest that single nucleotide polymorphisms within *FADS2* and/or *FASD1* genes are an important determinant of LC*n*-3 fatty acid status (Koletzko et al., 2011; Rzehak et al., 2009). Furthermore, the final synthesis of DHA requires β-oxidation within peroxisomes, and heritable polymorphisms in peroxisomal (*PEX*) genes are associated with peripheral and central DHA deficits and neuodevelopmental perturbations (Martinez et al., 1992). In healthy subjects residing in western countries, ALA→EPA biosynthesis is limited and ALA→DHA and EPA→DHA biosynthesis is negligible (Brenna et al., 2009). However, preformed EPA and DHA can be obtained directly from the diet, particularly from fatty cold water fish, including salmon, trout, tuna, as well as fish oil and algal-derived LC*n*-3 fatty acid supplements. Bypassing microsomal- and peroxisomal-mediated biosynthesis with preformed DHA is significantly more effective than ALA for increasing DHA composition in red blood cells (RBC) (Barceló-Coblijn et al., 2008), breast milk (Francois et al., 2003; Jensen et al., 2000) and cortical gray matter (Lin et al., 2011; Su et al., 1999; *see also* Figure 1). Therefore, LC*n*-3 fatty acid status is ultimately governed by gene-diet interactions.

An individual's LC*n*-3 fatty acid status can be determined using the fatty acid composition of RBC membranes by gas chromatography, and RBC LC*n*-3 fatty acid levels are a valid index of habitual dietary LC*n*-3 fatty acid intake (Fekete et al., 2009). For example, controlled LC*n*-3 fatty acid intervention studies have found that fish oil supplementation dose-dependently increases RBC LC*n*-3 fatty acid levels in human subjects (Barceló-Coblijn et al., 2008). Moreover, the greater annual fish and seafood consumption in Japan (148 lb/person) compared with the U.S. (48 lb/person)(WHO, 1996) is associated with a ~2-fold greater RBC membrane EPA+DHA composition in healthy Japanese adults (8.5±1.8%)(Itomura et al., 2008) compared with healthy U.S. adults (4.9±2.1%)(Sands et al., 2005). It is relevant therefore that cross-national epidemiological studies have found that higher per capita intake of fish/seafood is associated with lower lifetime prevalence rates of unipolar and bipolar depression (Hibbeln, 1998, Noaghiul & Hibbeln, 2003; Peet, 2004). Moreover, population studies have found that lower LC*n*-3 fatty acid intake is associated with increased risk for developing depressive symptoms (Astorg et al., 2008; Colangelo et al., 2009; Murakami et al., 2010; Raeder et al., 2007; Tanskanen et al., 2001; Timonen et al., 2004). Furthermore, prospective surveillance studies have found that low baseline LC*n*-3 fatty acid status is a predictor of suicide in MDD patients (Sublette et al., 2006) as well as treatment-emergent depression in human subjects receiving interferon-α (Lotrich et al., 2013; Su et al., 2010). Together, these data suggest that lower habitual dietary LC*n*-3 fatty acid intake and status may be associated with an elevated risk for mood dysregulation.

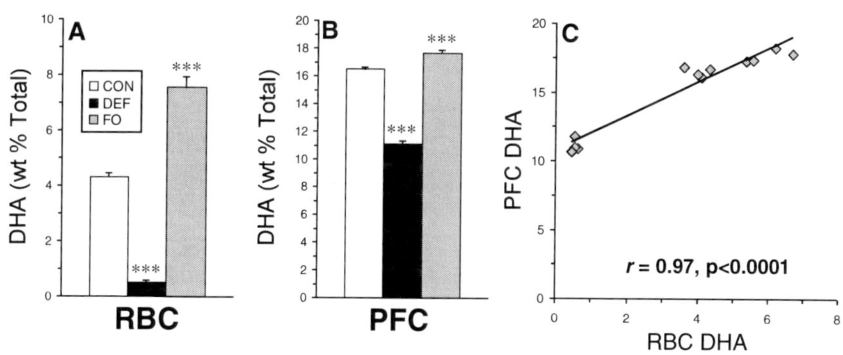

Figure 1. Adult RBC (A) and PFC (B) DHA levels (weight % total fatty acids) in rats fed a control diet (CON) containing 4.9% ALA, a diet containing no *n*-3 fatty acids (DEF), or a diet fortified with fish oil (FO) containing LC*n*-3 fatty acids (2.2% EPA, 1.7% DHA) during peri-adolescent development (postnatal day 21-90). Note that dietary *n*-3 fatty acid depletion is associated with significant RBC and PFC DHA deficits in young adulthood, and the fortifying the diet with LC*n*-3 fatty acids is associated with significant greater increases in RBC and PFC DHA levels in young adulthood compared with CON rats. Note also that among all rats RBC and PFC DHA levels are positively correlated (C). Values are group means ± S.E.M. ***$p \leq 0.0001$ *vs.* Controls.

Several independent studies from different countries have observed significant RBC membrane LC*n*-3 fatty acid deficits in MDD patients compared with healthy controls. A recent meta-analysis of 14 case-control studies found significant deficits in EPA and DHA in MDD patients (Lin et al., 2010). In bipolar patients, three independent studies have observed significant erythrocyte LC*n*-3 deficits compared with healthy controls (Chiu et al., 2003; McNamara et al., 2010c; Ranjekar et al., 2003). Importantly, RBC LC*n*-3 fatty acid deficits have also been observed in pediatric and adolescent patients with MDD or bipolar disorder (Clayton et al., 2008; Pottala et al., 2012). Moreover, medication-naïve first-episode psychotic patients exhibit RBC DHA deficits compared with healthy controls (Khan et al., 2002; Reddy et al., 2004), and a recent meta-analysis of 18 case-control studies observed significant DHA deficits in schizophrenic patients (Hoen et al., 2013). Lastly, case-control fatty acid composition studies have found that pediatric and adult ADHD patients exhibit RBC DHA deficits compared with healthy controls (Chen et al., 2004; Colter et al., 2008; Stevens et al., 1995; Young et al., 2004). Together, these case-control studies provide evidence that different psychiatric disorders are characterized by low LC*n*-3 fatty acid status which coincide with, and may precede, the initial onset of psychopathology.

Non-human primate cortical biopsy (Connor et al., 1990) and human postmortem brain (Carver et al., 2001) studies suggest that RBC and PFC DHA levels are positively correlated under steady state dietary conditions, though RBC DHA levels change more rapidly than PFC levels in response to changes in dietary LC*n*-3 fatty acid intake. Moreover, we have demonstrated that dietary *n*-3 fatty acid intake during adolescence is an important determinant of rat PFC and RBC DHA levels in young adulthood and that RBC and PFC DHA levels are positively correlated (Figure 1). A growing number of case-control studies have investigated the fatty acid composition of postmortem frontal gray matter from patients with mood and psychotic disorders. Some studies have observed lower LC*n*-3 fatty acid levels (McNamara et al., 2007a, 2007b, 2008a; Tatebayashi et al., 2013; Conlkin et al., 2010) while others have not (Igarashi et al., 2010; Lalovic et al., 2007; Yao et al., 2000), and a number of important extraneous variables, including medication effects and methodological limitations may account for this discrepancy (McNamara & Jandacek, 2011). Nevertheless, we reported that young adult patients with MDD (McNamara et al., 2007a), bipolar disorder (McNamara et al., 2008a), and schizophrenia (McNamara et al., 2007b) exhibit significant PFC DHA deficits compared with controls. While these postmortem findings must be viewed with caution, they are in general agreement with the RBC data and suggest that psychopathology may be associated with deficits in PFC DHA accrual.

While the etiology of LC*n*-3 fatty acid deficits observed in psychiatric patients is likely multifactorial (McNamara, 2013c), dietary LC*n*-3 fatty acid supplementation has been found to significantly increase patient RBC LC*n*-3 fatty acid levels (Amminger et al., 2010; Clayton et al., 2009; Wozniak et al., 2007). This observation indicates that LC*n*-3 fatty acid deficits in psychiatric patients are modifiable by increasing dietary LC*n*-3 fatty acid intake. Importantly, meta-analyses of controlled trials have observed a significant advantage of LC*n*-3 fatty acid supplementation over placebo for reducing depressive symptoms in patients with MDD (Appleton et al., 2010; Freeman et al., 2006; Lin & Su, 2007) or bipolar disorder (Sarris et al., 2012). Moreover, preliminary trials have found that LC*n*-3 fatty acid supplementation significantly reduces depression and manic symptom severity in pediatric and adolescent patients (Clayton et al., 2009; Nemets et al., 2006; Wozniak et al., 2007). Accumulating evidence also suggests that LC*n*-3 fatty acid supplementation may be efficacious for the treatment of positive and negative symptoms in patients with or at ultra-high risk for developing schizophrenia (Amminger et al., 2010; Emsley et al., 2002; Mellor et al., 1995; Peet et al., 2001), and for reducing attention deficits in pediatric and adolescent ADHD patients (Bloch et al., 2011). While this body of evidence suggests that low LC*n*-3 fatty acid status may represent a modifiable risk factor for psychopathology, the central mechanisms mediating this relationship remain poorly understood.

Role of DHA in PFC Development

Mammalian brain tissue is predominantly composed of lipids (60-65% of brain dry weight) which are comprised of saturated, monounsaturated, and polyunsaturated fatty acids. The principal LC*n*-3 polyunsaturated fatty acid found in mammalian PFC gray matter is DHA, which comprises approximately 10-20% of total fatty acid composition in the adult PFC (Carver et al., 2001; Connor et al., 1990; McNamara et al., 2008b). Although the omega-3 fatty acid precursors of DHA, including α-linolenic acid (ALA, 18:3*n*-3), EPA (20:5*n*-3), and docosapentaenoic acid (22:5*n*-3), cross the blood-brain barrier, they are rapidly oxidized (Chen et al., 2009) and consequently comprise <1% of total brain fatty acid composition (Carver et al., 2001). Unesterified DHA diffuses from plasma to brain at a rate that is equilibrated with brain DHA consumption (Ouellet et al., 2009; Rapoport et al., 2011), and preferentially accumulates in gray matter synaptasomal and mitochondrial membranes (Suzuki et al., 1997). DHA is mobilized from membrane phospholipids by the calcium-independent phospholipase A_2 ($iPLA_2$) isoform (Farooqui & Harrocks, 2004) and free DHA has been found to interact with second messenger signaling pathways associated with synaptic neurotransmission and plasticity (McNamara et al., 2006). It has been estimated that approximately 2-8% of rat brain DHA is replaced daily due to metabolism, and has a loss half-life in total rat brain phospholipids of 33 days under steady state ALA intake (DeMar et al., 2004; Rapoport et al., 2001). A preliminary tracer study estimated that the DHA half-life in healthy human brain phospholipids is 2.5 years (Umhau et al., 2009). Importantly, dietary *n*-3 fatty acid insufficiency is associated with reductions in $iPLA_2$ expression and activity in rat PFC (Rao et al., 2007a), and a >2-fold reduction in the loss half-life of DHA (Demar et al., 2004). Unlike the developing rat brain, following adolescent maturation brain DHA levels appear to become more resistance to turnover and loss in response to dietary *n*-3 fatty acid insufficiency (Bourre et al., 1992).

In the human brain DHA accumulates at a rapid rate during the third trimester *in utero*, and increases to approximately 9% of total fatty acid composition in term-birth infants (Clandinin et al., 1980a; Martinez & Mougan, 1998). Infants born preterm exhibit lower postmortem cortical DHA concentrations relative to term infants maintained on the same ALA-fortified formula (Clandinin et al., 1980a; Farquharson et al., 1992,1995; Martinez & Mougan, 1998). Similarly, non-human primates born preterm exhibit lower postmortem brain DHA concentrations relative to term-born primates whose mothers were maintained on the same diet (Sarkadi-Nagi et al., 2003,2004). Postnatally, PFC DHA composition continues to increase in a rapid a linear manner during childhood and adolescence, and stabilizes at approximately 15% of total fatty acid composition by ~20 years of age in subjects residing in the U.S. (Carver et al., 2001). In a preliminary postmortem study, we also found that DHA composition increases sharply in the PFC during normal human adolescent development, and that this increase is significantly blunted in young adult suicide victims (Figure 2). These postmortem findings suggest that the human PFC is associated with a linear increase in DHA composition during the childhood and adolescent period coinciding with rapid changes in PFC structural and functional maturation.

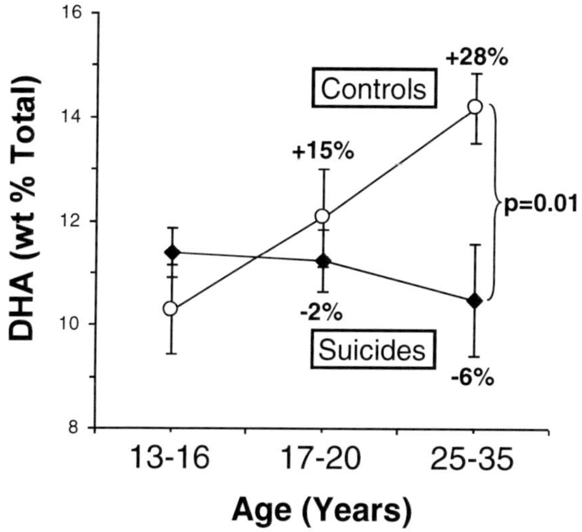

Figure 2. Comparison of DHA levels (weight % total fatty acids) in the human postmortem PFC (BA10) of typically developing adolescents and young adults and suicide victims (n=8-12/age group). Note that DHA levels progressively increase in the PFC of typically developing adolescents but not in suicide victims. Values are group means ± S.E.M.

During perinatal rat brain development, cortical DHA concentrations also increase sharply in parallel with active periods of neurogenesis, neuroblast migration, and synaptogenesis (Green & Yavin, 1996). Dietary-induced deficits in brain DHA accrual during perinatal maturation are associated with reductions in neurotrophic factor expression (Ikemoto et al., 2000; Rao et al., 2007b), neurite outgrowth (Calderon & Kim, 2004; Ikemoto et al., 1997), neurogenesis and migration (Beltz et al., 2007; Kawakita et al., 2006; Yavin et al., 2009), dendritic arborization (Sakamoto et al., 2007), embryonic cortical plate expansion (Coti Bertrand et al., 2006), and synaptogenesis and synaptic plasticity (Cao et al., 2009). Dietary-induced deficits in rat brain DHA accrual during perinatal maturation are also associated with neuronal shrinkage in limbic structures including the hippocampus (Ahmad et al., 2002). It is relevant, therefore, that postmortem histological studies have observed significant neuronal shrinkage in the PFC of patients with bipolar disorder and MDD (Cotter et al., 2005). Moreover, deficits in perinatal brain DHA accrual are associated with reductions in astrocyte-specific glucose transporter (GLUT1) expression and glucose uptake in the rat PFC (Pifferi et al., 2005; Ximenes da Silva et al., 2002), and postmortem histological studies found that young patients with mood disorders or schizophrenia exhibit elevated indices of astrocyte pathology in the PFC (Miguel-Hidalgo et al., 2000; Rajakowska et al., 2002). Lastly, deficits in PFC DHA accrual are associated with elevated pro-inflammatory signaling molecules in the rat PFC (Rao et al., 2007a), and histological studies have observed elevated pro-inflammatory signaling molecules in the postmortem PFC of bipolar disorder patients (Kim et al., 2011).

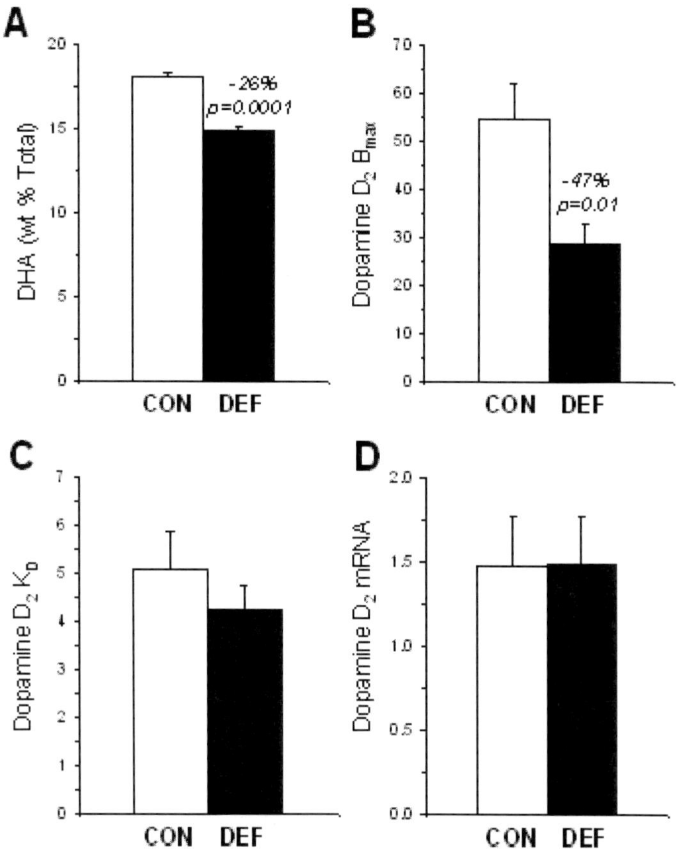

Figure 3. Effects of dietary n-3 fatty acid (ALA) depletion initiated prior to adolescence (postnatal day 21-90) on DHA levels (A), dopamine D_2 receptor binding density (B_{max})(B), dopamine D_2 receptor binding affinity (K_D)(C), and dopamine D_2 receptor mRNA expression (D) in the young adult PFC. Note that dietary n-3 fatty acid insufficiency and associated PFC DHA deficits are associated with lower dopamine D_2 receptor binding density in the young adulthood rat PFC. Values are group means ± S.E.M.

Cortical DHA accrual during perinatal rat brain development is required for the normal functional maturation of multiple neurotransmitter systems implicated in the pathophysiology and treatment of psychiatric disorders including dopamine and serotonin (Chalon, 2006). Specifically, perinatal deficits in PFC DHA accrual are associated with significant reductions in dopamine D_2 receptor binding in the young adult rat PFC (Delion et al., 1996; Zimmer et al., 2002). Our group has additionally found that dietary-induced deficits in PFC DHA accrual initiated prior to the adolescent period is sufficient to significantly reduce dopamine D_2 receptor binding density, but not binding affinity or mRNA expression, in the young adult PFC (Figure 3). From a functional perspective, preclinical *in vivo* microdialysis studies have found that perinatal deficits in brain DHA accrual are associated with enduring impairments in tyramine- and amphetamine-induced increases in extracellular dopamine levels in the adult rat PFC (Kodas et al., 2002; Zimmer et al., 1998, 2000, 2002). Histological studies have found that perinatal deficits in brain DHA accrual are associated reductions in dopamine neurons in the ventral tegmentum which projects dopamine axons to the PFC (Ahmad et al., 2008). Together, these preclinical findings suggest that perinatal deficits in brain DHA accrual are associated with significant impairments in mesocortical dopamine neurotransmission. It is relevant therefore that a postmortem study found that schizophrenic patients exhibit deficits in dopaminergic markers in the PFC consistent with impaired mesocortical dopamine function (Akil et al., 1999), and deficits in mesocortical dopamine transmission have long been thought to play a role in the pathophysiology and treatment of ADHD (Ernst et al., 1998; Rosa Neto et al., 2002; Swanson et al., 2006).

Pharmacological studies provide additional evidence for effects of perinatal deficits in cortical DHA accrual on dopamine-mediated behavior. Specifically, perinatal deficits in PFC DHA accrual are associated with significant decrements in haloperidol-induced catalepsy (Levant et al., 2004), which is mediated in part by PFC D_2 receptors (Lipska et al., 1995). Perinatal deficits in rat brain DHA accrual are also associated with augmented locomotor activity in response to acute amphetamine injection (Levant et al., 2004), and we found that even small dietary-induces reductions in PFC DHA levels are sufficient to augment amphetamine-induced behavioral sensitization in adult mice (McNamara et al., 2008c,d). Importantly, prepulse inhibition, a form of sensory gating that is modulated in part by PFC dopamine and predictive of amphetamine sensitization (Peleg-Raibstein et al., 2013), is significantly reduced by dietary-induced deficits in mouse brain DHA composition (Fedorova et al., 2009). Our group has additionally found that dietary-induced deficits in rat PFC DHA accrual initiated prior to the adolescent period is sufficient to significantly augment amphetamine-induced behavioral sensitization in young adult rats, and additionally found that this augmented response was associated with reduced dopamine turnover in the PFC (Figure 4). Interestingly, a neuroimaging study found that MDD patients exhibit a blunted PFC response following an amphetamine challenge (Tremblay et al., 2005), and chronic exposure to psychostimulants, followed by a prolonged abstinence period, is associated with PFC hypoactivation and reductions in PFC gray and white matter volumes (Fein et al., 2002; Fraklin et al., 2002; Lim et al., 2002; London et al., 2000; Tanabe et al., 2009).

Several lines of clinical and postmortem evidence have implicated abnormalities in PFC serotonin neurotransmission in the pathophysiology and treatment of MDD (Arango et al., 2002; Austin et al., 2002; Owens and Nemeroff, 1994). Preclinical studies have found that perinatal dietary *fortification* with LC*n*-3 fatty acids increase serotonin concentrations in rat PFC (Chalon et al., 1998), attenuate reductions in PFC 5-HT content in response to chronic stress (Vancassel et al., 2008), and decrease depression-like behavior in the forced swim test (Carlezon et al., 2005; Huang et al., 2008; Lakhwani et al., 2007). Conversely, perinatal deficits in cortical DHA accrual are associated with impaired fenfluramine-induced serotonin neurotransmission (Kodas et al., 2004) and increase aggression and depression-like behavior in the forced swim test (DeMar et al., 2006). It is relevant that MDD patients exhibit blunted fenfluramine-induced glucose metabolism in the PFC (Anderson et al., 2004). Moreover, perinatal deficits in cortical DHA accrual are associated with significant elevations in 5-HT_{2A} receptor binding density in the rat PFC (Delion et al., 1996), and elevated 5-HT_{2A} receptor binding density is observed in the postmortem PFC of depressed suicides (Arango et al., 1990; Pandey et al., 2002).

Clinical neurochemical studies have found that plasma LC*n*-3 fatty acid levels are positively correlated with cerebrospinal fluid (CSF) concentrations of the serotonin metabolite 5-hydroxyindoleacetic acid (5-HIAA) in healthy subjects (Hibbeln et al., 1998), and that low CSF 5-HIAA content is associated with suicidal behavior (Placidi et al., 2001). Furthermore, medication-free MDD patients exhibit significant elevations in internal jugular venoarterial 5-HIAA plasma content (Barton et al., 2008), and chronic treatment with selective serotonin reuptake inhibitors (SSRI) significantly decrease CSF and jugular venoarterial 5-HIAA content in depressed patients (Barton et al., 2008; Lundmark et al., 1994; Sheline et al., 1997). Perinatal deficits in cortical DHA accrual significantly increase 5-HIAA content in the young adult PFC

(McNamara et al., 2009a), and chronic SSRI treatment significantly decreases 5-HIAA content in the young adult PFC (McNamara et al., 2010b; Unceta et al., 2007). Collectively, these translational findings suggest that LC*n*-3 fatty acid deficiency during perinatal develop can lead to enduring alterations in PFC serotonin neurotransmission that are opposite to those produced by SSRI antidepressant medications.

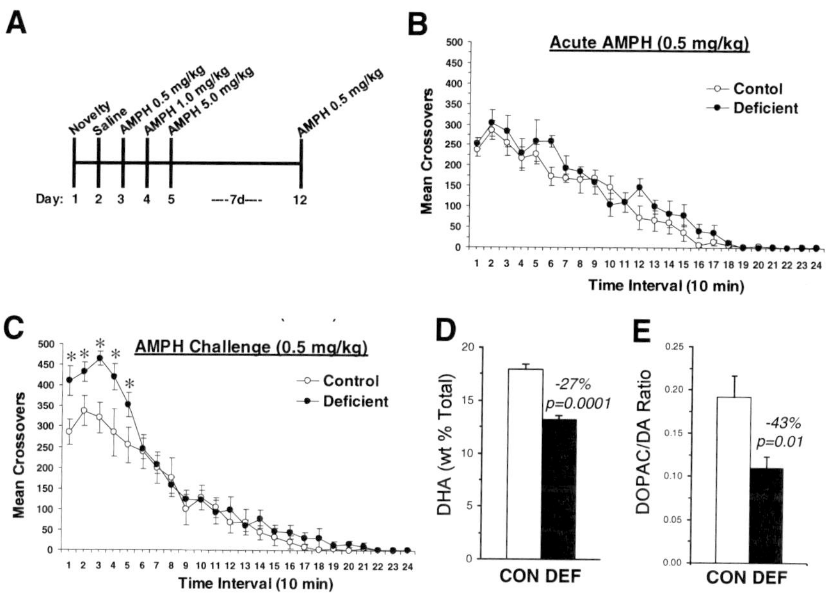

Figure 4. Effects of dietary *n*-3 fatty acid insufficiency during adolescence (postnatal day 21-90) on amphetamine (AMPH)-induced behavioral (locomotor activity) sensitization and dopamine metabolism in the young adulthood rat PFC. The escalating AMPH dose schedule is presented in (A). In response to acute low-dose AMPH (0.5 mg/kg), rats fed the control diet (*n*-3 fatty acid fortified, n=8) and *n*-3 fatty acid deficient diet (n=8) exhibit similar elevations in locomotor activity (B). Following treatment with escalating AMPH doses, low-dose AMPH (0.5 mg/kg) induces significantly greater locomotor activity in rats fed the *n*-3 fatty acid depleted diet compared with controls (C). PFC DHA levels are presented in (D) and PFC dopamine metabolism (dihydroxyphenylacetic acid (DOPAC)/dopamine (DA) ratio) determined immediately following the AMPH challenge is presented in (E). Values are group means ± S.E.M. $*p \leq 0.05$ *vs.* Controls.

In addition to neurotrophic effects, emerging evidence suggests that dietary LC*n*-3 fatty acid supplementation resulting in elevations in cortical DHA content is neuroprotective against a variety of cortical insults associated with oxidative stress, including focal and global ischemia (Belayev et al., 2009; Blondeau et al., 2002), glutamate excitotoxicity (Green et al., 2001; Hogyes et al., 2003; Ozyurt et al., 2007), traumatic head injury (Wu et al., 2004), and other neurotoxic agents (Meydan et al., 2012; Zararsiz et al., 2006). Dietary-induced elevations in brain DHA content prevent or attenuate neuropathological features in transgenic mice overexpressing the human APPswe gene, including dendritic pathology and plaque burden (Cole & Frautschy, 2006; Green et al., 2007; Hashimoto et al., 2005; Lim et al., 2005). Moreover, greater cortical DHA levels are associated with increased resilience of axons and white matter in experimental injury and inflammation models (Bailes et al., 2010; Tuzun et al., 2012; Ward et al., 2010). The mechanisms mediating the neuroprotective effects of DHA, and its lipoxygenase metabolite Neuroprotectin D1, may involve several complementary pathways including reductions in proinflammatory signaling, up-regulating antiapoptotic genes (*Bcl-2, Bcl-xl, Bfl-1*), and decreasing pro-apoptotic genes (*Bax, Bad*)(Bazan, 2009). These findings take on additional significance in view of postmortem data demonstrating elevated markers of excitotoxicity in the PFC of patients with bipolar disorder (Rao et al., 2010), and MRI studies finding that patients with psychiatric disorders exhibit reductions in PFC gray and white matter volumes (see below).

Clinical Neuroimaging Studies

Evidence from cross-sectional MRI studies have observed deficits in PFC structural and functional integrity in patients with MDD (Bora et al., 2012; Drevets, 2000; Sacher et al., 2012), bipolar disorder (Schneider et al., 2012; Strakowski et al., 2012), schizophrenia (De Peri et al., 2012; Vita et al., 2013), and ADHD (Castellanos et al., 2002; Helpern et al., 2011; Shaw & Rabin, 2009). The PFC has reciprocal connections with anterior temporal lobe structures including the amygdala mediated in part by the uncinate fasciculus white matter bundle (Figure 5) which gate amygdala outputs to the hypothalamus and nucleus accumbens (Ebeling & Von Cramon, 1992; Kier et al., 2004). Moreover, deficits in PFC white matter volume and structural integrity have been observed early in course of illness in patients with MDD (Cullen et al., 2010; Guo et al., 2012), bipolar disorder (Adler et al., 2006; Bellani & Brambilla, 2011; Lin et al., 2011), schizophrenia (Colombo et al., 2012), and ADHD (Silk et al., 2009). While is not known whether these deficits in PFC gray and white matter are associated with lower DHA status, or are preventable or reversible by increasing dietary DHA supplementation, emerging evidence from multimodal MRI studies suggest that there is a positive association between LC*n*-3 fatty acid status and cortical structural and functional integrity (McNamara, 2013a).

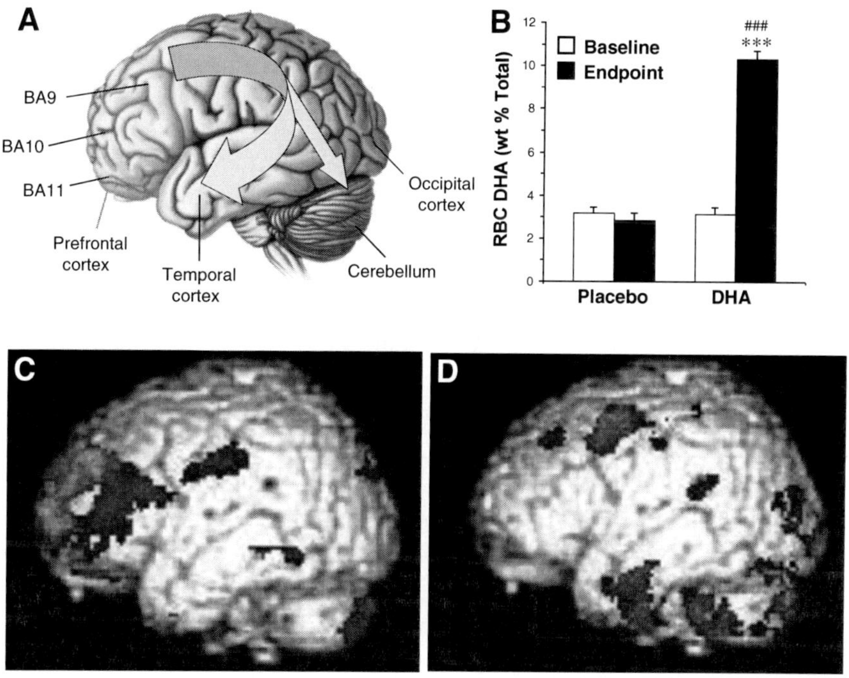

Figure 5. (A) Diagram illustrating the human PFC and major subdivisions (BA9 - DLPFC, BA10 - orbitofrontal cortex, BA11 - ventrolateral PFC) and the white matter bundles (i.e., uncinate fasciculus) linking the PFC with temporal lobe structures and the cerebellum (arrows). (B) RBC membrane DHA composition of healthy male children (aged 8-10 years) treated with placebo (n=10) or DHA (1200 mg/d, n=13) at baseline and study endpoint (8 weeks). Functional *t*-maps illustrating group (placebo vs. DHA) differences in baseline-to-endpoint change in regional activation (positive BOLD, DHA > placebo) (C) and deactivation (negative BOLD, placebo > DHA)(D) during performance of a sustained attention task (CPT-IP). The color gradient (red → yellow) reflects increasing statistical significance relative to placebo ($P \leq 0.05$ threshold and $T \leq 25$ cluster volume). Note that subjects receiving DHA exhibit greater baseline-to endpoint increases in PFC activity and greater baseline-to-endpoint decreases in temporal cortex and cerebellum activity compared with subjects receiving placebo. In (B) values are group mean ± S.E.M. $^{***}P \leq 0.001$ vs. baseline, $^{\#\#\#}P \leq 0.001$ vs. placebo at endpoint.

A positive relationship between DHA status during development and cortical structural integrity is suggested by structural MRI studies finding that children/adolescents born preterm, which is associated with early deficits in cortical DHA accrual (Clandinin et al., 1980a; Farquharson et al., 1992,1995; Martinez & Mougan, 1998), exhibit significant reductions in regional cortical and striatal gray matter volumes, reduced amygdala and hippocampal volumes, and reduced white matter volumes compared with age- and sex-matched term born controls (Peterson et al., 2000). It is also relevant that preterm children are at increased risk for developing ADHD (Bhutta et al., 2002; Cherkes-Julkowski, 1998), and that structural MRI studies have found that ADHD children exhibit patterns of cortical gray and white matter volume deficits similar to those observed in preterm children (Castellanos et al., 2002). Furthermore, intervention studies have found that postnatal dietary DHA supplementation improves visual attention processes in preterm infants (Carlson and Werkman, 1996). Pediatric patients with generalized peroxisomal disorders exhibit significant RBC and postmortem cortex DHA deficits (Martinez et al., 1995) and impaired myelinogenesis (Powers & Moser, 1998), and a preliminary structural MRI study found that treatment with DHA ethyl ester normalized or significantly increased brain white matter volumes in pediatric peroxisomal disorder patients (Martinez & Vazquez, 1998). However, a placebo-controlled structural MRI study found that postnatal DHA supplementation did not significantly alter age-related changes in white matter volume in premature infants (van Wezel-Meijler et al., 2002). A preliminary structural MRI study found that greater habitual intake of LC*n*-3 fatty acids was associated with larger gray matter volumes in the anterior cingulate cortex, the right hippocampus, and the right amygdala (Conklin et al., 2007). Together, these structural MRI findings provide preliminary support for a positive relationship between DHA status and cortical gray and white matter development.

In a controlled functional MRI trial, our group investigated the effects of 8-week DHA supplementation on cortical activity during performance of sustained attention task (CPT-IP) in healthy male children (McNamara et al., 2010a). At 8 weeks, erythrocyte membrane DHA composition increased significantly from baseline in subjects receiving DHA but not placebo (Figure 5B). During sustained attention, subjects receiving DHA exhibited significantly greater change from baseline in the activation of dorsolateral PFC (BA9), and greater decreases in the cerebellar cortex, relative to placebo. It is relevant therefore that mediation-naïve pediatric ADHD patients exhibit reduced PFC activation and greater cerebellar cortex activation while performing a sustained attention task (Rubia et al., 2009) a pattern that is opposite to that observed in healthy children following DHA supplmentation. Using a less stringent statistical threshold, greater increases in the PFC (Figure 5C) and greater decreases in temporal cortex (Figure 5D) were observed in the DHA group compared with placebo. Importantly, fMRI studies have found that mood disorders including MDD and bipolar disorder are associated with deficits in task-elicited PFC activation and greater activation in temporal lobe structures including the amygdala during emotional tasks (Anand et al., 2005; Altshuler et al., 2005). Together, these fMRI findings suggest that increasing DHA status during development augment PFC-regulated networks.

A positron emission tomography (PET) study using radiolabeled glucose ([^{18}F]-fluoro-2-deoxyglucose) evaluated the relationship between plasma DHA composition and resting state cerebral glucose metabolism in adult medication-free MDD patients (Sublette et al., 2009). Plasma DHA composition was positively correlated with glucose metabolism in the temporoparietal cortex, and negatively correlated with glucose metabolism in prefrontal cortex and anterior cingulate cortex. This study also found that plasma EPA levels were not significantly correlated with regional cerebral glucose metabolism. These preliminary PET data suggest that DHA status is correlated with regional cortical glucose metabolic activity, and that DHA status may have opposing effects on resting activity in the PFC and temporal cortex. In our fMRI study (McNamara et al., 2010a), we found that erythrocyte DHA composition was positively correlated with PFC activation during sustained attention. Together these findings suggest that blood DHA status is negatively associated with *resting* metabolic activity and positively associated with *functional* activity in the human PFC.

Proton magnetic resonance spectroscopy (^{1}H MRS) is a voxel-based technique that determines *in vivo* cortical concentrations of different chemical associated with cortical integrity and metabolism. For example, *myo*-inositol (mI) is metabolized from glucose via 1L-*myo*-inositol 1-phosphate synthase and is predominantly concentrated in astroctyes, and *N*-acetyl aspartate (NAA) is primarily localized to neurons and is positively correlated with mitochondrial metabolism (Brand et al., 1993; Griffin et al., 2002). ^{1}H MRS studies have consistently observed lower NAA concentrations in human cortical infarcts during the acute or subacute phase of ischemia (Lanfermann et al., 1995). In a preclinical ^{1}H MRS study, our group investigated the effects of perinatal and postnatal deficits in DHA accrual on mI and NAA concentrations in rat medial prefrontal cortex. We found that perinatal, but not postnatal, deficits in brain DHA accrual were associated with reductions in mI, but not

NAA, concentrations in the rat PFC (McNamara et al., 2009b). Additionally, acute treatment with a selective agonist at dopamine D_1 phosphoinositide-coupled receptors increased mI concentrations in the perinatal deficiency group but not in controls (McNamara et al., 2009b). In a clinical ^{1}H MRS study employing healthy developing male children, we recently found that subjects with low RBC DHA status exhibited lower mI and NAA concentrations in the anterior cingulate cortex compared with subjects in the high RBC DHA status group (McNamara et al., 2013b). A preliminary placebo-controlled ^{1}H MRS study found that 12-week supplementation with EPA selectively increased NAA concentrations in the anterior cingulate cortex of medicated patients with bipolar disorder (Frangou et al., 2007). Although preliminary, these ^{1}H MRS data are consistent with DHA status being positively associated with cortical markers of neuronal (NAA) and astrocyte (mI) integrity.

CONCLUSION

There is now considerable evidence that major psychiatric disorders are associated with peripheral and potentially central LC*n*-3 fatty acid deficits and reductions in PFC structure and function evident early in the course of illness. Moreover, psychiatric disorders frequently initially emerge during adolescence, a period associated with rapid increases in PFC DHA levels as well as dynamic changes in PFC structural maturation. As proof-of-concept, preclinical studies have demonstrated that dietary-induced deficits in cortical DHA accrual during perinatal development lead to enduring deficits in PFC biochemistry and neuropathological features, including neuronal shrinkage and deficits in astrocyte mediated glucose uptake, that recapitulate findings in the postmortem PFC of psychiatric patients. Preliminary human neuroimaging studies also suggest that LC*n*-3 fatty acid status is positively associated with cortical gray and white matter volumes as well as PFC functional activity. Together, this body of translational evidence supports the proposition that low LC*n*-3 fatty acid status during active periods of PFC maturation may represent a modifiable risk factor for deficits in PFC structure and function and associated psychopathology. However, direct support for this pathoetiological mechanism will require evidence that increasing LC*n*-3 fatty acid status can prevent progressive PFC gray and white matter volume deficits and associated psychopathology in human patients. Such studies are currently feasible and are supported by the finding that increasing LC*n*-3 fatty acid status prevented or delayed the initial onset of psychosis in ultra-high risk adolescents (Amminger et al., 2010).

REFERENCES

Adler CM, Adams J, DelBello MP, Holland SK, Schmithorst V, Levine A, Jarvis K, Strakowski SM. Evidence of white matter pathology in bipolar disorder adolescents experiencing their first episode of mania: a diffusion tensor imaging study. *Am J Psychiatry.* 2006;163:322-324.

Ahmad A, Moriguchi T, Salem N. Decrease in neuron size in docosahexaenoic acid-deficient brain. *Pediatr Neurol.* 2002;26:210-218.

Ahmad SO, Park JH, Radel JD, Levant B. Reduced numbers of dopamine neurons in the substantia nigra pars compacta and ventral tegmental area of rats fed an n-3 polyunsaturated fatty acid-deficient diet: a stereological study. *Neurosci Lett.* 2008;438:303-307.

Akil M, Pierri JN, Whitehead RE, Edgar CL, Mohila C, Sampson AR, Lewis DA. Lamina-specific alterations in the dopamine innervation of the prefrontal cortex in schizophrenic subjects. *Am J Psychiatry.* 1999;156:1580-1589.

Altshuler L, Bookheimer S, Proenza MA, Townsend J, Sabb F, Firestine A, Bartzokis G, Mintz J, Mazziotta J, Cohen MS. Increased amygdala activation during mania: a functional magnetic resonance imaging study. *Am J Psychiatry.* 2005;162:1211-1213.

Amminger GP, Schäfer MR, Papageorgiou K, Klier CM, Cotton SM, Harrigan SM, Mackinnon A, McGorry PD, Berger GE. Long-chain omega-3 fatty acids for indicated prevention of psychotic disorders: a randomized, placebo-controlled trial. *Arch Gen Psychiatry.* 2010;67:146-154.

Anand A, Li Y, Wang Y, Wu J, Gao S, Bukhari L, Mathews VP, Kalnin A, Lowe MJ. Activity and connectivity of brain mood regulating circuit in depression: a functional magnetic resonance study. *Biol Psychiatry.* 2005;57:1079-1088.

Anderson AD, Oquendo MA, Parsey RV, Milak MS, Campbell C, Mann JJ. Regional brain responses to serotonin in major depressive disorder. *J Affect Disord.* 2004;82:411-417.

Angst F, Stassen HH, Clayton PJ, Angst J. Mortality of patients with mood disorders: follow-up over 34-38 years. *J Affect Disord.* 2002;68:167-181.

Appleton KM, Rogers PJ, Ness AR. Updated systematic review and meta-analysis of the effects of n-3 long-chain polyunsaturated fatty acids on depressed mood. *Am J Clin Nutr*. 2010;91:757-770.

Arango V, Ernsberger P, Marzuk PM, Chen JS, Tierney H, Stanley M, Reis DJ, Mann JJ. Autoradiographic demonstration of increased serotonin 5-HT2 and beta-adrenergic receptor binding sites in the brain of suicide victims. *Arch. Gen. Psychiatry*. 1990;47:1038-1047.

Arango V, Underwood MD, Mann JJ. Serotonin brain circuits involved in major depression and suicide. *Prog. Brain. Res*. 2002;136:443-453.

Astorg P, Couthouis A, Bertrais S, Arnault N, Meneton P, Guesnet P, Alessandri JM, Galan P, Hercberg S. Association of fish and long-chain n-3 polyunsaturated fatty acid intakes with the occurrence of depressive episodes in middle-aged French men and women. *Prostaglandins Leukot Essent Fatty Acids*. 2008;78:171-182.

Austin MC, Whitehead RE, Edgar CL, Janosky JE, Lewis DA. Localized decrease in serotonin transporter-immunoreactive axons in the prefrontal cortex of depressed subjects committing suicide. *Neuroscience*. 2002;114:807-815.

Ayuso-Gutierrez JL, del Rio Vega JM. Factors influencing relapse in the long-term course of schizophrenia. *Schizophr Res*. 1997;28:199-206.

Bailes JE, Mills JD. Docosahexaenoic acid reduces traumatic axonal injury in a rodent head injury model. *J Neurotrauma*. 2010;27:1617-1624.

Barceló-Coblijn G, Murphy EJ, Othman R, Moghadasian MH, Kashour T, Friel JK. Flaxseed oil and fish-oil capsule consumption alters human red blood cell n-3 fatty acid composition: a multiple-dosing trial comparing 2 sources of n-3 fatty acid. *Am J Clin Nutr*. 2008;88:801-809.

Barton DA, Esler MD, Dawood T, Lambert EA, Haikerwal D, Brenchley C, Socratous F, Hastings J, Guo L, Wiesner G, Kaye DM, Bayles R, Schlaich MP, Lambert GW. Elevated brain serotonin turnover in patients with depression: effect of genotype and therapy. *Arch Gen Psychiatry*. 2008;65:38-46.

Bazan NG. Cellular and molecular events mediated by docosahexaenoic acid-derived neuroprotectin D1 signaling in photoreceptor cell survival and brain protection. *Prostaglandins Leukot Essent Fatty Acids*. 2009;81:205-211.

Belayev L, Khoutorova L, Atkins KD, Bazan NG. Robust docosahexaenoic acid-mediated neuroprotection in a rat model of transient, focal cerebral ischemia. *Stroke*. 2009;40:3121-3126.

Bellani M, Brambilla P. Diffusion imaging studies of white matter integrity in bipolar disorder. *Epidemiol Psychiatr Sci.* 2011;20:137-140.

Beltz BS, Tlusty MF, Benton JL, Sandeman DC. Omega-3 fatty acids upregulate adult neurogenesis. Neurosci Lett. 2007;415:154-158.

Bhutta AT, Cleves MA, Casey PH, Cradock MM, Anand KJ. Cognitive and behavioral outcomes of school-aged children who were born preterm: a meta-analysis. *JAMA* 2002;288:728-737.

Bloch MH, Qawasmi A. Omega-3 fatty acid supplementation for the treatment of children with attention-deficit/hyperactivity disorder symptomatology: systematic review and meta-analysis. *J Am Acad Child Adolesc Psychiatry.* 2011;50:991-1000.

Blondeau N, Widmann C, Lazdunski M, Heurteaux C. Polyunsaturated fatty acids induce ischemic and epileptic tolerance. *Neuroscience.* 2002;109:231-241.

Bora E, Fornito A, Pantelis C, Yücel M. Gray matter abnormalities in Major Depressive Disorder: a meta-analysis of voxel based morphometry studies. *J Affect Disord.* 2012;138:9-18.

Bourre JM, Dumont OS, Piciotti MJ, Pascal GA, Durand GA. Dietary alpha-linolenic acid deficiency in adult rats for 7 months does not alter brain docosahexaenoic acid content, in contrast to liver, heart and testes. *Biochim Biophys Acta.* 1992;1124:119-122.

Brand, A., C. Richter-Landsberg, and D. Leibfritz. Multinuclear NMR studies on the energy metabolism of glial and neuronal cells. *Dev. Neurosci.* 1993;15:289-298.

Brenna JT, Salem N Jr, Sinclair AJ, Cunnane SC; International Society for the Study of Fatty Acids and Lipids, ISSFAL. alpha-Linolenic acid supplementation and conversion to n-3 long-chain polyunsaturated fatty acids in humans. *Prostaglandins Leukot Essent Fatty Acids.* 2009;80:85-91.

Brown S. Excess mortality of schizophrenia. A meta-analysis. *Br J Psychiatry.* 1997;171:502-508.

Burke KC, Burke JD Jr, Rae DS, Regier DA. Comparing age at onset of major depression and other psychiatric disorders by birth cohorts in five US community populations. *Arch Gen Psychiatry.* 1991;48:789-795.

Calderon F, Kim HY. Docosahexaenoic acid promotes neurite growth in hippocampal neurons. *J Neurochem.* 2004;90:979-988.

Cao D, Kevala K, Kim J, Moon HS, Jun SB, Lovinger D, Kim HY. Docosahexaenoic acid promotes hippocampal neuronal development and synaptic function. *J Neurochem.* 2009;111:510-521.

Carlezon WA Jr, Mague SD, Parow AM, Stoll AL, Cohen BM, Renshaw PF. Antidepressant-like effects of uridine and omega-3 fatty acids are potentiated by combined treatment in rats. *Biol. Psychiatry*. 2005;57:343-350.

Carlson SE, Werkman SH. A randomized trial of visual attention of preterm infants fed docosahexaenoic acid until two months. *Lipids*. 1996;31:85-90.

Carver JD, Benford VJ, Han B, Cantor AB. The relationship between age and the fatty acid composition of cerebral cortex and erythrocytes in human subjects. *Brain Res Bull*. 2001;56:79-85.

Castellanos FX, Lee PP, Sharp W, Jeffries NO, Greenstein DK, Clasen LS, Blumenthal JD, James RS, Ebens CL, Walter JM, Zijdenbos A, Evans AC, Giedd JN, Rapoport JL. Developmental trajectories of brain volume abnormalities in children and adolescents with attention-deficit/hyperactivity disorder. *JAMA*. 2002;288:1740-1748.

Cavanagh J, Smyth R, Goodwin GM. Relapse into mania or depression following lithium discontinuation: a 7-year follow-up. *Acta Psychiatr Scand*. 2004;109:91-95.

Chalon S, Delion-Vancassel S, Belzung C, Guilloteau D, Leguisquet AM, Besnard JC, Durand G. Dietary fish oil affects monoaminergic neurotransmission and behavior in rats. *J. Nutr*. 1998;128:2512-2519.

Chalon S. Omega-3 fatty acids and monoamine neurotransmission. *Prostaglandins Leukot Essent Fatty Acids*. 2006;75:259-269.

Chen CT, Liu Z, Ouellet M, Calon F, Bazinet RP. Rapid beta-oxidation of eicosapentaenoic acid in mouse brain: an in situ study. *Prostaglandins Leukot Essent Fatty Acids*. 2009;80:157-163.

Chen JR, Hsu SF, Hsu CD, Hwang LH, Yang SC. Dietary patterns and blood fatty acid composition in children with attention-deficit hyperactivity disorder in Taiwan. *J. Nutr. Biochem*. 2004;15:467-472.

Cherkes-Julkowski M. Learning disability, attention-deficit disorder, and language impairment as outcomes of prematurity: a longitudinal descriptive study. *J Learn Disabil*. 1998;31:294-306.

Chiu CC, Huang SY, Su KP, Lu ML, Huang MC, Chen CC, Shen WW. Polyunsaturated fatty acid deficit in patients with bipolar mania. *Eur Neuropsychopharmacol*. 2003;13:99-103.

Clandinin MT, Chappell JE, Leong S, Heim T, Swyer PR, Chance GW. Extrauterine fatty acid accretion in infant brain: implications for fatty acid requirements. *Early Hum Dev*. 1980a;4:131-138.

Clandinin MT, Chappell JE, Leong S, Heim T, Swyer PR, Chance GW. Intrauterine fatty acid accretion rates in human brain: implications for fatty acid requirements. *Early Hum Dev.* 1980b;4:121-129.

Clayton EH, Hanstock TL, Hirneth SJ, Kable CJ, Garg ML, Hazell PL. Long-chain omega-3 polyunsaturated fatty acids in the blood of children and adolescents with juvenile bipolar disorder. *Lipids.* 2008;43:1031-1038.

Clayton EH, Hanstock TL, Hirneth SJ, Kable CJ, Garg ML, Hazell PL. Reduced mania and depression in juvenile bipolar disorder associated with long-chain omega-3 polyunsaturated fatty acid supplementation. *Eur J Clin Nutr.* 2009;63:1037-1040.

Colangelo LA, He K, Whooley MA, Daviglus ML, Liu K. Higher dietary intake of long-chain omega-3 polyunsaturated fatty acids is inversely associated with depressive symptoms in women. *Nutrition.* 2009;25:1011-1019.

Cole GM, Frautschy SA. Docosahexaenoic acid protects from amyloid and dendritic pathology in an Alzheimer's disease mouse model. *Nutr Health* 2006;18:249-59.

Colombo RR, Schaufelberger MS, Santos LC, Duran FL, Menezes PR, Scazufca M, Busatto GF, Zanetti MV. Voxelwise evaluation of white matter volumes in first-episode psychosis. *Psychiatry Res.* 2012;202:198-205.

Colter AL, Cutler C, Meckling KA. Fatty acid status and behavioural symptoms of attention deficit hyperactivity disorder in adolescents: a case-control study. *Nutr J.* 2008;7:8.

Conklin SM, Gianaros PJ, Brown SM, Yao JK, Hariri AR, Manuck SB, Muldoon MF. Long-chain omega-3 fatty acid intake is associated positively with corticolimbic gray matter volume in healthy adults. *Neurosci Lett.* 2007;421:209-212.

Conklin SM, Runyan CA, Leonard S, Reddy RD, Muldoon MF, Yao JK. Age-related changes of n-3 and n-6 polyunsaturated fatty acids in the anterior cingulate cortex of individuals with major depressive disorder. *Prostaglandins Leukot Essent Fatty Acids.* 2010;82:111-119.

Connor WE, Neuringer M, Lin DS. Dietary effects on brain fatty acid composition: the reversibility of n-3 fatty acid deficiency and turnover of docosahexaenoic acid in the brain, erythrocytes, and plasma of rhesus monkeys. *J Lipid Res.* 1990;31:237-247.

Coti Bertrand P, O'Kusky JR, Innis SM. Maternal dietary (n-3) fatty acid deficiency alters neurogenesis in the embryonic rat brain. *J Nutr.* 2006;136:1570-1575.

Cotter D, Hudson L, Landau S. Evidence for orbitofrontal pathology in bipolar disorder and major depression, but not in schizophrenia. *Bipolar Disord.* 2005;7:358-369.

Cullen KR, Klimes-Dougan B, Muetzel R, Mueller BA, Camchong J, Houri A, Kurma S, Lim KO. Altered white matter microstructure in adolescents with major depression: a preliminary study. *J Am Acad Child Adolesc Psychiatry*. 2010;49:173-183.

De Peri L, Crescini A, Deste G, Fusar-Poli P, Sacchetti E, Vita A. Brain structural abnormalities at the onset of schizophrenia and bipolar disorder: a meta-analysis of controlled magnetic resonance imaging studies. *Curr Pharm Des*. 2012;18:486-494.

Delion S, Chalon S, Guilloteau D, Besnard JC, Durand G. alpha-Linolenic acid dietary deficiency alters age-related changes of dopaminergic and serotoninergic neurotransmission in the rat frontal cortex. *J. Neurochem.* 1996;66:1582-1591.

DeMar JC Jr, Ma K, Bell JM, Igarashi M, Greenstein D, Rapoport SI. One generation of n-3 polyunsaturated fatty acid deprivation increases depression and aggression test scores in rats. *J. Lipid. Res.* 2006;47:172-180.

DeMar JC Jr, Ma K, Bell JM, Rapoport SI. Half-lives of docosahexaenoic acid in rat brain phospholipids are prolonged by 15 weeks of nutritional deprivation of n-3 polyunsaturated fatty acids. *J. Neurochem.* 2004;91:1125-1137.

Drevets WC. Functional anatomical abnormalities in limbic and prefrontal cortical structures in major depression. *Prog Brain Res.* 2000;126:413-431.

Ebeling U, von Cramon D. Topography of the uncinate fascicle and adjacent temporal fiber tracts. *Acta Neurochir* (Wien). 1992;115:143-148.

Ehringer MA, Rhee SH, Young S, Corley R, Hewitt JK. Genetic and environmental contributions to common psychopathologies of childhood and adolescence: a study of twins and their siblings. *J. Abnorm. Child. Psychol*. 2006;34:1-17.

Emsley R, Myburgh C, Oosthuizen P, van Rensburg SJ. Randomized, placebo-controlled study of ethyl-eicosapentaenoic acid as supplemental treatment in schizophrenia. *Am. J. Psychiatry*. 2002;159:1596-1598.

Ernst M, Zametkin AJ, Matochik JA, Jons PH, Cohen RM. DOPA decarboxylase activity in attention deficit hyperactivity disorder adults. A [fluorine-18]fluorodopa positron emission tomographic study. *J. Neurosci.* 1998;18:5901-5907.

Farooqui AA, Horrocks LA. Brain phospholipases A2: a perspective on the history. *Prostaglandins Leukot Essent Fatty Acids* 2004;71:161-169.

Farquharson J, Cockburn F, Patrick WA, Jamieson EC, Logan RW. Infant cerebral cortex phospholipid fatty-acid composition and diet. *Lancet* 1992;340:810-813.

Farquharson J, Jamieson EC, Abbasi KA, Patrick WJ, Logan RW, Cockburn F. Effect of diet on the fatty acid composition of the major phospholipids of infant cerebral cortex. *Arch Dis Child.* 1995;72:198-203.

Fedorova I, Alvheim AR, Hussein N, Salem N Jr. Deficit in prepulse inhibition in mice caused by dietary n-3 fatty acid deficiency. *Behav Neurosci.* 2009;123:1218-1225.

Fein G, Di Sclafani V, Meyerhoff DJ. Prefrontal cortical volume reduction associated with frontal cortex function deficit in 6-week abstinent crack-cocaine dependent men. *Drug Alcohol Depend.* 2002;68:87-93.

Fekete K, Marosvölgyi T, Jakobik V, Decsi T. Methods of assessment of n-3 long-chain polyunsaturated fatty acid status in humans: a systematic review. *Am J Clin Nutr.* 2009;89:2070S-2084S.

Francois CA, Connor SL, Bolewicz LC, Connor WE. Supplementing lactating women with flaxseed oil does not increase docosahexaenoic acid in their milk. *Am J Clin Nutr.* 2003;77:226-233.

Frangou S, Lewis M, Wollard J, Simmons A. Preliminary in vivo evidence of increased N-acetyl-aspartate following eicosapentanoic acid treatment in patients with bipolar disorder. *J Psychopharmacol.* 2007;21:435-439.

Franklin TR, Acton PD, Maldjian JA, Gray JD, Croft JR, Dackis CA, O'Brien CP, Childress AR. Decreased gray matter concentration in the insular, orbitofrontal, cingulate, and temporal cortices of cocaine patients. *Biol Psychiatry.* 2002;51:134-142.

Freeman MP, Hibbeln JR, Wisner KL, Davis JM, Mischoulon D, Peet M, Keck PE Jr, Marangell LB, Richardson AJ, Lake J, Stoll AL. Omega-3 fatty acids: evidence basis for treatment and future research in psychiatry. *J. Clin. Psychiatry.* 2006;67:1954-1967.

Geddes JR, Carney SM, Davies C, Furukawa TA, Kupfer DJ, Frank E, Goodwin GM. Relapse prevention with antidepressant drug treatment in depressive disorders: a systematic review. *Lancet* 2003;361:653-661.

Giedd JN, Lalonde FM, Celano MJ, White SL, Wallace GL, Lee NR, Lenroot RK. Anatomical brain magnetic resonance imaging of typically developing children and adolescents. *J Am Acad Child Adolesc Psychiatry.* 2009;48:465-470.

Green KN, Martinez-Coria H, Khashwji H, Hall EB, Yurko-Mauro KA, Ellis L, LaFerla FM. Dietary docosahexaenoic acid and docosapentaenoic acid ameliorate amyloid-beta and tau pathology via a mechanism involving presenilin 1 levels. *J Neurosci.* 2007;27:4385-95.

Green P, Glozman S, Weiner L, Yavin E. Enhanced free radical scavenging and decreased lipid peroxidation in the rat fetal brain after treatment with ethyl docosahexaenoate. *Biochim Biophys Acta.* 2001;1532:203-212.

Green P, Yavin E. Fatty acid composition of late embryonic and early postnatal rat brain. *Lipids.* 1996;31:859-865.

Greenberg PE, Kessler RC, Birnbaum HG, Leong SA, Lowe SW, Berglund PA, Corey-Lisle PK. The economic burden of depression in the United States: how did it change between 1990 and 2000? *J Clin Psychiatry.* 2003;64:1465-1475.

Griffin, J. L., M. Bollard, J. K. Nicholson, and K. Bhakoo. Spectral profiles of cultured neuronal and glial cells derived from HRMAS (1)H NMR spectroscopy. *NMR Biomed.* 2002;15:375-384.

Guo WB, Liu F, Xue ZM, Gao K, Wu RR, Ma CQ, Liu ZN, Xiao CQ, Chen HF, Zhao JP. Altered white matter integrity in young adults with first-episode, treatment-naive, and treatment-responsive depression. *Neurosci Lett.* 2012;522:139-144.

Hashimoto M, Hossain S, Agdul H, Shido O. Docosahexaenoic acid-induced amelioration on impairment of memory learning in amyloid beta-infused rats relates to the decreases of amyloid beta and cholesterol levels in detergent-insoluble membrane fractions. *Biochim Biophys Acta.* 2005;1738:91-98.

Helpern JA, Adisetiyo V, Falangola MF, Hu C, Di Martino A, Williams K, Castellanos FX, Jensen JH. Preliminary evidence of altered gray and white matter microstructural development in the frontal lobe of adolescents with attention-deficit hyperactivity disorder: a diffusional kurtosis imaging study. *J Magn Reson Imaging.* 2011;33:17-23.

Hibbeln JR, Linnoila M, Umhau JC, Rawlings R, George DT, Salem N Jr. Essential fatty acids predict metabolites of serotonin and dopamine in cerebrospinal fluid among healthy control subjects, and early- and late-onset alcoholics. *Biol. Psychiatry.* 1998;44:235-242.

Hibbeln JR. Fish consumption and major depression. *Lancet* 1998;351:1213.

Hoen WP, Lijmer JG, Duran M, Wanders RJ, van Beveren NJ, de Haan L. Red blood cell polyunsaturated fatty acids measured in red blood cells and schizophrenia: A meta-analysis. *Psychiatry Res.* 2013 [Epub ahead of print]

Högyes E, Nyakas C, Kiliaan A, Farkas T, Penke B, Luiten PG. Neuroprotective effect of developmental docosahexaenoic acid supplement against excitotoxic brain damage in infant rats. *Neuroscience.* 2003;119:999-1012.

Huang SY, Yang HT, Chiu CC, Pariante CM, Su KP. Omega-3 fatty acids on the forced-swimming test. *J. Psychiatr. Res.* 2008;42:58-63.

Igarashi M, Ma K, Gao F, Kim HW, Greenstein D, Rapoport SI, Rao JS. Brain lipid concentrations in bipolar disorder. *J Psychiatr Res.* 2010;44:177-182.

Ikemoto A, Kobayashi T, Watanabe S, Okuyama H. Membrane fatty acid modifications of PC12 cells by arachidonate or docosahexaenoate affect neurite outgrowth but not norepinephrine release. *Neurochem Res.* 1997;22:671-678.

Ikemoto A, Nitta A, Furukawa S, Ohishi M, Nakamura A, Fujii Y, Okuyama H. Dietary n-3 fatty acid deficiency decreases nerve growth factor content in rat hippocampus. *Neurosci Lett.* 2000;285:99-102.

Itomura M, Fujioka S, Hamazaki K, Kobayashi K, Nagasawa T, Sawazaki S, Kirihara Y, Hamazaki T. Factors influencing EPA+DHA levels in red blood cells in Japan. *In Vivo.* 2008;22:131-135.

Jensen CL, Maude M, Anderson RE, Heird WC. Effect of docosahexaenoic acid supplementation of lactating women on the fatty acid composition of breast milk lipids and maternal and infant plasma phospholipids. *Am J Clin Nutr.* 2000;71:292S-299S.

Kawakita E, Hashimoto M, Shido O. Docosahexaenoic acid promotes neurogenesis in vitro and in vivo. *Neuroscience.* 2006;139:991-997.

Kessler RC, Berglund P, Demler O, Jin R, Merikangas KR, Walters EE. Lifetime prevalence and age-of-onset distributions of DSM-IV disorders in the National Comorbidity Survey Replication. *Arch Gen Psychiatry.* 2005;62:593-602.

Kessler RC, Merikangas KR, Wang PS. Prevalence, comorbidity, and service utilization for mood disorders in the United States at the beginning of the twenty-first century. *Annu Rev Clin Psychol.* 2007;3:137-158.

Khan MM, Evans DR, Gunna V, Scheffer RE, Parikh VV, Mahadik SP. Reduced erythrocyte membrane essential fatty acids and increased lipid peroxides in schizophrenia at the never-medicated first-episode of psychosis and after years of treatment with antipsychotics. *Schizophr. Res.* 2002;58:1-10.

Kier EL, Staib LH, Davis LM, Bronen RA. MR imaging of the temporal stem: anatomic dissection tractography of the uncinate fasciculus, inferior occipitofrontal fasciculus, and Meyer's loop of the optic radiation. *AJNR Am J Neuroradiol.* 2004;25:677-691.

Kim HW, Rapoport SI, Rao JS. Altered arachidonic acid cascade enzymes in postmortem brain from bipolar disorder patients. *Mol Psychiatry.* 2011;16:419-428.

Kleinman L, Lowin A, Flood E, Gandhi G, Edgell E, Revicki D. Costs of bipolar disorder. *Pharmacoeconomics.* 2003;21:601-622.

Kodas E, Galineau L, Bodard S, Vancassel S, Guilloteau D, Besnard JC, Chalon S. Serotoninergic neurotransmission is affected by n-3 polyunsaturated fatty acids in the rat. *J. Neurochem.* 2004;89:695-702.

Kodas E, Vancassel S, Lejeune B, Guilloteau D, Chalon S. Reversibility of n-3 fatty acid deficiency-induced changes in dopaminergic neurotransmission in rats: critical role of developmental stage. *J. Lipid. Res.* 2002;43:1209-1219.

Koletzko B, Lattka E, Zeilinger S, Illig T, Steer C. Genetic variants of the fatty acid desaturase gene cluster predict amounts of red blood cell docosahexaenoic and other polyunsaturated fatty acids in pregnant women: findings from the Avon Longitudinal Study of Parents and Children. *Am J Clin Nutr.* 2011;93:211-219.

Lakhwani L, Tongia SK, Pal VS, Agrawal RP, Nyati P, Phadnis P. Omega-3 fatty acids have antidepressant activity in forced swimming test in Wistar rats. *Acta Pol Pharm.* 2007;64:271-276.

Lalovic A, Levy E, Canetti L, Sequeira A, Montoudis A, Turecki G. Fatty acid composition in postmortem brains of people who completed suicide. *J Psychiatry Neurosci.* 2007;32:363-370.

Lanfermann H, Kugel H, Heindel W, Herholz K, Heiss WD, Lackner K. Metabolic changes in acute and subacute cerebral infarctions: findings at proton MR spectroscopic imaging. *Radiology.* 1995;196:203-210.

Levant B, Radel JD, Carlson SE. Decreased brain docosahexaenoic acid during development alters dopamine-related behaviors in adult rats that are differentially affected by dietary remediation. *Behav. Brain. Res.* 2004;152:49-57.

Lim GP, Calon F, Morihara T, Yang F, Teter B, Ubeda O, Salem N Jr, Frautschy SA, Cole GM. A diet enriched with the omega-3 fatty acid docosahexaenoic acid reduces amyloid burden in an aged Alzheimer mouse model. *J Neurosci.* 2005;25:3032-40.

Lim KO, Choi SJ, Pomara N, Wolkin A, Rotrosen JP. Reduced frontal white matter integrity in cocaine dependence: a controlled diffusion tensor imaging study. *Biol Psychiatry.* 2002;51:890-895.

Lin F, Weng S, Xie B, Wu G, Lei H. Abnormal frontal cortex white matter connections in bipolar disorder: a DTI tractography study. *J Affect Disord.* 2011;131:299-306.

Lin PY, Huang SY, Su KP. A meta-analytic review of polyunsaturated fatty acid compositions in patients with depression. *Biol Psychiatry.* 2010;68:140-147.

Lin PY, Su KP. A meta-analytic review of double-blind, placebo-controlled trials of antidepressant efficacy of omega-3 fatty acids. *J Clin Psychiatry.* 2007;68:1056-1061.

Lin YH, Shah S, Salem N Jr. Altered essential fatty acid metabolism and composition in rat liver, plasma, heart and brain after microalgal DHA addition to the diet. *J Nutr Biochem.* 2011;22:758-765.

Lipska BK, Jaskiw GE, Braun AR, Weinberger DR. Prefrontal cortical and hippocampal modulation of haloperidol-induced catalepsy and apomorphine-induced stereotypic behaviors in the rat. *Biol. Psychiatry.* 1995;38:255-262.

London ED, Ernst M, Grant S, Bonson K, Weinstein A. Orbitofrontal cortex and human drug abuse: functional imaging. *Cereb Cortex.* 2000;10:334-342.

Lotrich FE, Sears B, McNamara RK. Elevated ratio of arachidonic acid to long-chain omega-3 fatty acids predicts depression development following interferon-alpha treatment: Relationship with interleukin-6. *Brain Behav Immun.* 2013 [Epub ahead of print].

Lundmark J, Wålinder J, Alling C, Manniche PM, Dalgaard L. The effect of paroxetine on cerebrospinal fluid concentrations of neurotransmitter metabolites in depressed patients. *Eur Neuropsychopharmacol.* 1994;4:1-6.

Martínez M, Mougan I. Fatty acid composition of human brain phospholipids during normal development. *J. Neurochem.* 1998;71:2528-2533.

Martinez M, Vazquez E. MRI evidence that docosahexaenoic acid ethyl ester improves myelination in generalized peroxisomal disorders. *Neurology.* 1998;51:26-32.

Martinez M. Abnormal profiles of polyunsaturated fatty acids in the brain, liver, kidney and retina of patients with peroxisomal disorders. *Brain Res.* 1992; 583:171-182.

Martinez M. Polyunsaturated fatty acids in the developing human brain, erythrocytes and plasma in peroxisomal disease: therapeutic implications. *J Inherit Metab Dis.* 1995;8:61-75.

McGuffin P, Owen MJ, Gottesman II., Eds Psychiatric Genetics & Genomics (revised) Oxford: Oxford University Press; 2004.

McNamara RK, Ostrander M, Abplanalp W, Richtand NM, Benoit SC, Clegg DJ. Modulation of phosphoinositide-protein kinase C signal transduction by omega-3 fatty acids: implications for the pathophysiology and treatment of recurrent neuropsychiatric illness. *Prostaglandins Leukot Essent Fatty Acids.* 2006;75:237-257.

McNamara RK, Hahn C-G, Jandacek R, Rider T, Tso P, Stanford K, Richtand NM. Selective deficits in the omega-3 fatty acid docosahexaenoic acid in the postmortem orbitofrontal cortex of patients with major depressive disorder. *Biol Psychiatry* 2007a;62:17-24.

McNamara RK, Jandacek R, Rider T, Tso P, Richtand NM, Stanford K. Abnormalities in the fatty acid composition of the postmortem orbitofrontal cortex of schizophrenic patients: Gender differences and partial normalization with antipsychotic medications. *Schizophr Res.* 2007b;91:37-50.

McNamara RK, Jandacek R, Rider T, Tso P, Stanford K, Hahn C-G, Richtand NM. Deficits in docosahexaenoic acid and associated elevations in the metabolism of arachidonic acid and saturated fatty acids in the postmortem orbitofrontal cortex of patients with bipolar disorder. *Psychiatric Res.* 2008a;160:285-299.

McNamara RK, Liu Y, Jandacek R, Rider T, Tso P. The aging human orbitofrontal cortex: Decreasing polyunsaturated fatty acid composition and associated increases in lipogenic gene expression and stearoyl-CoA desaturase activity. *Prostaglandins Leukot Essent Fatty Acids* 2008b;78:293-304.

McNamara RK, Sullivan J, Richtand NM, Jandacek R, Rider T, Tso P, Campbell N, Lipton JW. Omega-3 fatty acid deficiency augments amphetamine-induced behavioral sensitization in adult DBA/2J mice: Relationship with ventral striatum dopamine concentrations. *Synapse* 2008c;62:725-735.

McNamara RK, Sullivan J, Richtand NM. Omega-3 fatty acid deficiency augments amphetamine-induced behavioral sensitization in adult mice: Prevention by chronic lithium treatment. *J Psychiatric Res.* 2008d;42:458-468.

McNamara RK, Able J, Liu Y, Jandacek R, Rider T, Tso P, Lipton JW. Omega-3 fatty acid deficiency during perinatal development increases serotonin turnover in the prefrontal cortex and decreases midbrain tryptophan hydroxylase-2 expression in adult female rats: dissociation from estrogenic effects. *J Psychiatr Res.* 2009a;43:656-663.

McNamara RK, Able JA, Jandacek R, Rider T, Tso P, Lindquist DM. Perinatal omega-3 fatty acid deficiency selectively reduces myo-inositol levels in the adult rat prefrontal cortex: An in vivo ^{1}H-MRS study. *J Lipid Res.* 2009b;50:405-411.

McNamara RK, Able JA, Jandacek R, Rider T, Tso P, Eliassen J, Alfieri D, Weber W, Jarvis K, DelBello MP, Strakowski SM, Adler CM. Docosahexaenoic acid supplementation increases prefrontal cortex activation during sustained attention in healthy boys: A placebo-controlled, dose-ranging, functional magnetic resonance imaging study. *Am J Clin Nutr.* 2010a;91:1060-1067.

McNamara RK, Able JA, Rider T, Tso P, Jandacek R. Effect of chronic fluoxetine treatment on male and female rat erythrocyte and prefrontal cortex fatty acid composition. Prog *Neuropsychopharmacol Biol Psychiatry.* 2010b;34:1317-1321.

McNamara RK, Jandacek R, Rider T, Tso P, Dwivedi Y, Pandey GN. Selective deficits in erythrocyte docosahexaenoic acid composition in adult patients with bipolar disorder and major depressive disorder. *J Affect Disord.* 2010c;126:303-311.

McNamara RK, Jandacek R. Investigation of postmortem brain polyunsaturated fatty acid composition in psychiatric disorders: Limitations, challenges, and future directions. *J Psychiatry Res.* 2011;45:44-46.

McNamara RK. Deciphering the role of docosahexaenoic acid in brain maturation and pathology with magnetic resonance imaging. *Prostaglandins Leukot Essent Fatty Acids.* 2013a;88:33-42.

McNamara RK, Jandacek R, Rider T, Tso P, Weber W, Chu W-J, Strakowski SM, Adler CM, DelBello MP. Low docosahexaenoic acid status is associated with reduced indices of cortical integrity in the anterior cingulate of healthy boys: A ^{1}H MRS study. *Nutr Neurosci.* 2013b; [Epub ahead of print].

McNamara RK. Long-Chain Omega-3 Fatty Acid Deficiency in Mood Disorders: Rationale for Treatment and Prevention. *Curr Drug Discov Technol.* 2013c; [Epub ahead of print].

Mellor JE, Laugharne JD, Peet M. Schizophrenic symptoms and dietary intake of n-3 fatty acids. *Schizoph. Res. 1995;18:85-86.*

Meydan S, Altas M, Nacar A, Ozturk OH, Tas U, Zararsiz I, Sarsilmaz M. The protective effects of omega-3 fatty acid against toluene-induced neurotoxicity in prefrontal cortex of rats. *Hum Exp Toxicol.* 2012;31:1179-1185.

Meyers J, Classi P, Wietecha L, Candrilli S. Economic burden and comorbidities of attention-deficit/hyperactivity disorder among pediatric patients hospitalized in the United States. *Child Adolesc Psychiatry Ment Health.* 2010;4:31.

Miguel-Hidalgo JJ, Baucom C, Dilley G, Overholser JC, Meltzer HY, Stockmeier CA, Rajkowska G. Glial fibrillary acidic protein immunoreactivity in the prefrontal cortex distinguishes younger from older adults in major depressive disorder. *Biol Psychiatry.* 2000;48:861-873.

Murakami K, Miyake Y, Sasaki S, Tanaka K, Arakawa M. Fish and n-3 polyunsaturated fatty acid intake and depressive symptoms: Ryukyus Child Health Study. *Pediatrics.* 2010 Sep;126(3):e623-30.

Nemets H, Nemets B, Apter A, Bracha Z, Belmaker RH. Omega-3 treatment of childhood depression: a controlled, double-blind pilot study. *Am J Psychiatry.* 2006;163:1098-1100.

Noaghiul S, Hibbeln JR. Cross-national comparisons of seafood consumption and rates of bipolar disorders. *Am J Psychiatry.* 2003;160:2222-2227.

Osby U, Brandt L, Correia N, Ekbom A, Sparén P. Excess mortality in bipolar and unipolar disorder in Sweden. *Arch Gen Psychiatry.* 2001;58:844-850.

Ouellet M, Emond V, Chen CT, Julien C, Bourasset F, Oddo S, LaFerla F, Bazinet RP, Calon F. Diffusion of docosahexaenoic and eicosapentaenoic acids through the blood-brain barrier: An in situ cerebral perfusion study. *Neurochem Int.* 2009;55:476-482.

Owens MJ, Nemeroff CB. Role of serotonin in the pathophysiology of depression: focus on the serotonin transporter. *Clin. Chem.* 1994;40:288-295.

Ozyurt B, Sarsilmaz M, Akpolat N, Ozyurt H, Akyol O, Herken H, Kus I. The protective effects of omega-3 fatty acids against MK-801-induced neurotoxicity in prefrontal cortex of rat. *Neurochem Int.* 2007;50:196-202.

Pandey GN, Dwivedi Y, Rizavi HS, Ren X, Pandey SC, Pesold C, Roberts RC, Conley RR, Tamminga CA. Higher expression of serotonin 5-HT(2A) receptors in the postmortem brains of teenage suicide victims. *Am. J. Psychiatry.* 2002;159:419-429.

Peet M, Brind J, Ramchand CN, Shah S, Vankar GK. Two double-blind placebo-controlled pilot studies of eicosapentaenoic acid in the treatment of schizophrenia. *Schizophr Res.* 2001;49:243-251.

Peet M. International variations in the outcome of schizophrenia and the prevalence of depression in relation to national dietary practices: an ecological analysis. *Br J Psychiatry* 2004;184:404-408.

Peleg-Raibstein D, Hauser J, Lopez LH, Feldon J, Gargiulo PA, Yee BK. Baseline prepulse inhibition expression predicts the propensity of developing sensitization to the motor stimulant effects of amphetamine in C57BL/6 mice. *Psychopharmacology* (Berl). 2013;225:341-352.

Perlis RH, Dennehy EB, Miklowitz DJ, Delbello MP, Ostacher M, Calabrese JR, Ametrano RM, Wisniewski SR, Bowden CL, Thase ME, Nierenberg AA, Sachs G. Retrospective age at onset of bipolar disorder and outcome during two-year follow-up: results from the STEP-BD study. *Bipolar Disord.* 2009;11:391-400.

Peterson BS, Vohr B, Staib LH, Cannistraci CJ, Dolberg A, Schneider KC, Katz KH, Westerveld M, Sparrow S, Anderson AW, Duncan CC, Makuch RW, Gore JC, Ment LR. Regional brain volume abnormalities and long-term cognitive outcome in preterm infants. *JAMA* 2000;284:1939-1947.

Pifferi F, Roux F, Langelier B, Alessandri JM, Vancassel S, Jouin M, Lavialle M, Guesnet P. (n-3) polyunsaturated fatty acid deficiency reduces the expression of both isoforms of the brain glucose transporter GLUT1 in rats. *J Nutr.* 2005;135:2241-2246.

Placidi GP, Oquendo MA, Malone KM, Huang YY, Ellis SP, Mann JJ. Aggressivity, suicide attempts, and depression: relationship to cerebrospinal fluid monoamine metabolite levels. *Biol Psychiatry.* 2001;50:783-791.

Pottala JV, Talley JA, Churchill SW, Lynch DA, von Schacky C, Harris WS. Red blood cell fatty acids are associated with depression in a case-control study of adolescents. Prostaglandins Leukot Essent *Fatty Acids.* 2012;86:161-165.

Powers JM, Moser HW. Peroxisomal disorders: genotype, phenotype, major neuropathologic lesions, and pathogenesis. *Brain Pathol.* 1998;8:101-120.

Raeder MB, Steen VM, Vollset SE, Bjelland I. Associations between cod liver oil use and symptoms of depression: the Hordaland Health Study. *J Affect Disord* 2007;101:245-249.

Rajkowska G, Miguel-Hidalgo JJ, Makkos Z, Meltzer H, Overholser J, Stockmeier C. Layer-specific reductions in GFAP-reactive astroglia in the dorsolateral prefrontal cortex in schizophrenia. *Schizophr Res.* 2002;57:127-138.

Ranjekar PK, Hinge A, Hegde MV, Ghate M, Kale A, Sitasawad S, Wagh UV, Debsikdar VB, Mahadik SP. Decreased antioxidant enzymes and membrane essential polyunsaturated fatty acids in schizophrenic and bipolar mood disorder patients. *Psychiatry Res.* 2003;121:109-122.

Rao JS, Ertley RN, DeMar JC Jr, Rapoport SI, Bazinet RP, Lee HJ. Dietary n-3 PUFA deprivation alters expression of enzymes of the arachidonic and docosahexaenoic acid cascades in rat frontal cortex. *Mol. Psychiatry.* 2007a;12:151-157.

Rao JS, Ertley RN, Lee HJ, DeMar JC Jr, Arnold JT, Rapoport SI, Bazinet RP. n-3 polyunsaturated fatty acid deprivation in rats decreases frontal cortex BDNF via a p38 MAPK-dependent mechanism. *Mol Psychiatry.* 2007b;12:36-46.

Rao JS, Harry GJ, Rapoport SI, Kim HW. Increased excitotoxicity and neuroinflammatory markers in postmortem frontal cortex from bipolar disorder patients. *Mol Psychiatry.* 2010;15:384-392.

Rapoport SI, Chang MC, Spector AA. Delivery and turnover of plasma-derived essential PUFAs in mammalian brain. *J. Lipid Res.* 2001;42:678-685.

Rapoport SI, Ramadan E, Basselin M. Docosahexaenoic acid (DHA) incorporation into the brain from plasma, as an in vivo biomarker of brain DHA metabolism and neurotransmission. *Prostaglandins Other Lipid Mediat.* 2011;96:109-113.

Reddy RD, Keshavan MS, Yao JK. Reduced red blood cell membrane essential polyunsaturated fatty acids in first episode schizophrenia at neuroleptic-naive baseline. *Schizophr Bull.* 2004;30:901-911.

Rosa Neto P, Lou H, Cumming P, Pryds O, Gjedde A. Methylphenidate-evoked potentiation of extracellular dopamine in the brain of adolescents with premature birth: correlation with attentional deficit. *Ann.N. Y. Acad. Sci.* 2002;965:434-439.

Rubia K, Smith AB, Halari R, Matsukura F, Mohammad M, Taylor E, Brammer MJ. Disorder-specific dissociation of orbitofrontal dysfunction in boys with pure conduct disorder during reward and ventrolateral prefrontal dysfunction in boys with pure ADHD during sustained attention. *Am J Psychiatry.* 2009;166:83-94.

Rzehak P, Heinrich J, Klopp N, Schaeffer L, Hoff S, Wolfram G, Illig T, Linseisen J. Evidence for an association between genetic variants of the fatty acid desaturase 1 fatty acid desaturase 2 (FADS1 FADS2) gene cluster and the fatty acid composition of erythrocyte membranes. *Br J Nutr.* 2009;101:20-26.

Sacher J, Neumann J, Fünfstück T, Soliman A, Villringer A, Schroeter ML. Mapping the depressed brain: a meta-analysis of structural and functional alterations in major depressive disorder. *J Affect Disord.* 2012;140:142-148.

Sakamoto T, Cansev M, Wurtman RJ. Oral supplementation with docosahexaenoic acid and uridine-5'-monophosphate increases dendritic spine density in adult gerbil hippocampus. *Brain Res.* 2007;1182:50-59.

Sands SA, Reid KJ, Windsor SL, Harris WS. The impact of age, body mass index, and fish intake on the EPA and DHA content of human erythrocytes. *Lipids.* 2005;40:343-347.

Sarkadi-Nagy E, Wijendran V, Diau GY, Chao AC, Hsieh AT, Turpeinen A, Nathanielsz PW, Brenna JT. The influence of prematurity and long chain polyunsaturate supplementation in 4-week adjusted age baboon neonate brain and related tissues. *Pediatr. Res.* 2003;54:244-252.

Sarkadi-Nagy E, Wijendran V, Diau GY, Chao AC, Hsieh AT, Turpeinen A, Lawrence P, Nathanielsz PW, Brenna JT. Formula feeding potentiates docosahexaenoic and arachidonic acid biosynthesis in term and preterm baboon neonates. *J. Lipid. Res.* 2004;45:71-80.

Sarris J, Mischoulon D, Schweitzer I. Omega-3 for bipolar disorder: meta-analyses of use in mania and bipolar depression. *J Clin Psychiatry.* 2012;73:81-86.

Schneider MR, DelBello MP, McNamara RK, Strakowski SM, Adler CM. Neuroprogression in bipolar disorder. *Bipolar Disord.* 2012;14:356-374.

Shaw P, Rabin C. New insights into attention-deficit/hyperactivity disorder using structural neuroimaging. *Curr Psychiatry Rep.* 2009;11:393-398.

Sheline Y, Bardgett ME, Csernansky JG. Correlated reductions in cerebrospinal fluid 5-HIAA and MHPG concentrations after treatment with selective serotonin reuptake inhibitors. *J Clin Psychopharmacol.* 1997;17:11-14.

Silk TJ, Vance A, Rinehart N, Bradshaw JL, Cunnington R. White-matter abnormalities in attention deficit hyperactivity disorder: a diffusion tensor imaging study. *Hum Brain Mapp.* 2009;30:2757-2765.

Stevens LJ, Zentall SS, Deck JL, Abate ML, Watkins BA, Lipp SR, Burgess JR. Essential fatty acid metabolism in boys with attention-deficit hyperactivity disorder. *Am. J. Clin. Nutr.* 1995;62:761-768.

Strakowski SM, Adler CM, Almeida J, Altshuler LL, Blumberg HP, Chang KD, DelBello MP, Frangou S, McIntosh A, Phillips ML, Sussman JE, Townsend JD. The functional neuroanatomy of bipolar disorder: a consensus model. *Bipolar Disord.* 2012;14:313-325.

Su HM, Bernardo L, Mirmiran M, Ma XH, Corso TN, Nathanielsz PW, Brenna JT. Bioequivalence of dietary alpha-linolenic and docosahexaenoic acids as sources of docosahexaenoate accretion in brain and associated organs of neonatal baboons. *Pediatr Res.* 1999;45:87-93.

Su KP, Huang SY, Peng CY, Lai HC, Huang CL, Chen YC, Aitchison KJ, Pariante CM. Phospholipase A2 and cyclooxygenase 2 genes influence the risk of interferon-alpha-induced depression by regulating polyunsaturated fatty acids levels. *Biol Psychiatry.* 2010;67:550-557.

Sublette ME, Hibbeln JR, Galfalvy H, Oquendo MA, Mann JJ. Omega-3 polyunsaturated essential fatty acid status as a predictor of future suicide risk. *Am J Psychiatry.* 2006;163:1100-1102.

Sublette ME, Milak MS, Hibbeln JR, Freed PJ, Oquendo MA, Malone KM, Parsey RV, Mann JJ. Plasma polyunsaturated fatty acids and regional cerebral glucose metabolism in major depression. *Prostaglandins Leukot Essent Fatty Acids.* 2009;80:57-64.

Sullivan PF, Neale MC, Kendler KS. Genetic epidemiology of major depression: review and meta-analysis. *Am. J. Psychiatry.* 2000;157:1552-1562.

Suzuki H, Manabe S, Wada O, Crawford MA. Rapid incorporation of docosahexaenoic acid from dietary sources into brain microsomal, synaptosomal and mitochondrial membranes in adult mice. *Int. J. Vitam. Nutr. Res.* 1997;67:272-278.

Swanson CJ, Perry KW, Koch-Krueger S, Katner J, Svensson KA, Bymaster FP. Effect of the attention deficit/hyperactivity disorder drug atomoxetine on extracellular concentrations of norepinephrine and dopamine in several brain regions of the rat. *Neuropharmacology.* 2006;50:755-760.

Tanabe J, Tregellas JR, Dalwani M, Thompson L, Owens E, Crowley T, Banich M. Medial orbitofrontal cortex gray matter is reduced in abstinent substance-dependent individuals. *Biol Psychiatry.* 2009 15;65:160-164.

Tanskanen A, Hibbeln JR, Tuomilehto J, Uutela A, Haukkala A, Viinamäki H, Lehtonen J, Vartiainen E. Fish consumption and depressive symptoms in the general population in Finland. *Psychiatr Serv* 2001;52:529-531.

Tatebayashi Y, Nihonmatsu-Kikuchi N, Hayashi Y, Yu X, Soma M, Ikeda K. Abnormal fatty acid composition in the frontopolar cortex of patients with affective disorders. *Transl Psychiatry.* 2013.

Timonen M, Horrobin D, Jokelainen J, Laitinen J, Herva A, Räsänen P. Fish consumption and depression: the Northern Finland 1966 birth cohort study. *J Affect Disord* 2004;82:447-452.

Tremblay LK, Naranjo CA, Graham SJ, Herrmann N, Mayberg HS, Hevenor S, Busto UE. Functional neuroanatomical substrates of altered reward processing in major depressive disorder revealed by a dopaminergic probe. *Arch. Gen. Psychiatry*. 2005;62:1228-1236.

Tsuang M. Schizophrenia: genes and environment. *Biol Psychiatry*. 2000;47:210-220.

Tuzun F, Kumral A, Dilek M, Ozbal S, Ergur B, Yesilirmak DC, Duman N, Yılmaz O, Ozkan H. Maternal omega-3 fatty acid supplementation protects against lipopolysaccharide-induced white matter injury in the neonatal rat brain. *J Matern Fetal Neonatal Med*. 2012;25:849-854.

Umhau JC, Zhou W, Carson RE, Rapoport SI, Polozova A, Demar J, Hussein N, Bhattacharjee AK, Ma K, Esposito G, Majchrzak S, Herscovitch P, Eckelman WC, Kurdziel KA, Salem N Jr. Imaging incorporation of circulating docosahexaenoic acid into the human brain using positron emission tomography. *J Lipid Res*. 2009;50:1259-1268.

Unceta N, Barrondo S, Ruiz de Azúa I, Gómez-Caballero A, Goicolea MA, Sallés J, Barrio RJ. Determination of fluoxetine, norfluoxetine and their enantiomers in rat plasma and brain samples by liquid chromatography with fluorescence detection. *J Chromatogr B Analyt Technol Biomed Life Sci*. 2007;852:519-528.

van Wezel-Meijler G, van der Knaap MS, Huisman J, Jonkman EJ, Valk J, Lafeber HN. Dietary supplementation of long-chain polyunsaturated fatty acids in preterm infants: effects on cerebral maturation. *Acta Paediatr*. 2002;91:942-950.

Vancassel S, Leman S, Hanonick L, Denis S, Roger J, Nollet M, Bodard S, Kousignian I, Belzung C, Chalon S. n-3 polyunsaturated fatty acid supplementation reverses stress-induced modifications on brain monoamine levels in mice. *J Lipid Res*. 2008;49:340-348.

Vita A, De Peri L, Deste G, Sacchetti E. Progressive loss of cortical gray matter in schizophrenia: a meta-analysis and meta-regression of longitudinal MRI studies. *Transl Psychiatry*. 2013.

Ward RE, Huang W, Curran OE, Priestley JV, Michael-Titus AT. Docosahexaenoic acid prevents white matter damage after spinal cord injury. *J Neurotrauma*. 2010;27:1769-1780.

Wozniak J, Biederman J, Mick E, Waxmonsky J, Hantsoo L, Best C, Cluette-Brown JE, Laposata M. Omega-3 fatty acid monotherapy for pediatric bipolar disorder: a prospective open-label trial. *Eur Neuropsychopharmacol*. 2007;17:440-447.

Wu A, Ying Z, Gomez-Pinilla F. Dietary omega-3 fatty acids normalize BDNF levels, reduce oxidative damage, and counteract learning disability after traumatic brain injury in rats. *J Neurotrauma*. 2004;21:1457-1467.

Wu EQ, Birnbaum HG, Shi L, Ball DE, Kessler RC, Moulis M, Aggarwal J. The economic burden of schizophrenia in the United States in 2002. *J Clin Psychiatry*. 2005;66:1122-1129.

Ximenes da Silva A, Lavialle F, Gendrot G, Guesnet P, Alessandri JM, Lavialle M. Glucose transport and utilization are altered in the brain of rats deficient in n-3 polyunsaturated fatty acids. *J Neurochem*. 2002;81:1328-1337.

Yao JK, Leonard S, Reddy RD. Membrane phospholipid abnormalities in postmortem brains from schizophrenic patients. *Schizophr Res*. 2000;42:7-17.

Yavin E, Himovichi E, Eilam R. Delayed cell migration in the developing rat brain following maternal omega 3 alpha linolenic acid dietary deficiency. *Neuroscience*. 2009;162:1011-1122.

Young GS, Maharaj NJ, Conquer JA. Blood phospholipid fatty acid analysis of adults with and without attention deficit/hyperactivity disorder. *Lipids*. 2004;39:117-123.

Zararsiz I, Kus I, Akpolat N, Songur A, Ogeturk M, Sarsilmaz M. Protective effects of omega-3 essential fatty acids against formaldehyde-induced neuronal damage in prefrontal cortex of rats. *Cell Biochem Funct*. 2006;24:237-244.

Zimmer L, Hembert S, Durand G, Breton P, Guilloteau D, Besnard JC, Chalon S. Chronic n-3 polyunsaturated fatty acid diet-deficiency acts on dopamine metabolism in the rat frontal cortex: a microdialysis study. *Neurosci. Lett*. 1998;240:177-181.

Zimmer L, Delpal S, Guilloteau D, Aïoun J, Durand G, Chalon S. Chronic n-3 polyunsaturated fatty acid deficiency alters dopamine vesicle density in the rat frontal cortex. *Neurosci. Lett*. 2000;284:25-28.

Zimmer L, Vancassel S, Cantagrel S, Breton P, Delamanche S, Guilloteau D, Durand G, Chalon S. The dopamine mesocorticolimbic pathway is affected by deficiency in n-3 polyunsaturated fatty acids. *Am. J. Clin. Nutr*. 2002;75:662-667.

In: Prefrontal Cortex
Editors: R. O. Collins and J. L. Adams
ISBN 978-1-62618-663-7

Chapter 2

ADDICTION AND PREFRONTAL CORTEX

Eduardo López-Caneda and Úrsula Martínez
Department of Clinical Psychology and Psychobiology,
University of Santiago de Compostela, Galicia, Spain

ABSTRACT

Addiction is usually defined as the continued use of substances or activities despite their negative consequences. Different models have been proposed to explain why people start using drugs and why they still continue using even when they experience physical, psychological and/or social problems. In this context, prefrontal cortex (PFC), which has been involved in complex cognitive functions such as abstract thinking, planning, inhibitory control or decision-making, has gained much of the attention when explaining addiction due to its implication in different aspects related to addictives behaviours. In this chapter, we will focus on the PFC and its involvement in the addictives processes, paying particular attention to the somatic marker hypothesis. According to this model, substance abusers as well as patients with ventromedial prefrontal cortex (VMPC) lesions, show altered decision-making, characterized by a tendency to choose the immediate reward and by not taking into account long-term consequences of their behaviour. Growing scientific evidence indicates that core aspects of addiction may be explained in terms of an abnormal decision-making. The aim of this chapter is to review the previous literature regarding the role of the PFC in this process and, therefore, in the addictive behaviour. After describing the anatomy and functions of the PFC, different models and definitions of addiction will be discussed. Then, we will focus on the somatic marker model, which establishes that the altered decision-making in addiction is a consequence of an abnormal functioning of a distributed neural network critical for the processing of emotional information involving several regions of the PFC and limbic system. Accordingly, an examination of the scientific evidences that support the role of PFC in addiction will be conducted. Finally, we will discuss the implications for addiction treatment and prevention.

I. INTRODUCTION

One of the essential statements extracted from the work of Heraclitus (535 BC-475 BC), a Greek philosopher, was that "you cannot step twice into the same river". This is because of the continuous change that the river experiences as its waters never stop flowing or moving. In some sense, it can also be applied to the human beings who never wake up twice with the same brain, as it happened with the river of Heraclitus, human brain is always changing, or in the words of the philosopher in "perpetual flow".

Besides the changes that are naturally produced in the brain during the development, there are also changes which are "artificially" produced, i.e., changes that have no place in a natural way but are induced. Drugs are an example of externally induced changes in the brain. For example, through modifications of the action of chemical messengers in the brain (neurotransmitters), psychoactive substances can act on the nervous system of individuals changing not only their thoughts and behavior, but also the structure and configuration of the brain.

Although it is well known that drugs lead to brain abnormalities, the fact of whether these changes in brain structure and function are the cause of addictive behaviors or whether there is some grade of cerebral dysfunction preceding drug abuse is still a question that remains unanswered. But what we do know is that some individuals with drug dependence have a marked inability to evaluate the long-term consequences of their behavior which leads them to make decisions based only on the immediate benefit, without taking into account that these choices may be coupled with negative future consequences (for their health, social and/or working life etc.).

Different theories have emerged trying to explain the phenomenon of the addictive behaviors. From the neuroscience perspective, one of the theories that has gained much of the attention is the somatic marker hypothesis. According to this, which was originally proposed by Antonio Damasio [1], the decision-making process depends on the neural circuitry involved in emotions and feelings regulation. Under this model, some subjects with compulsive drug use would be similar to patients with ventromedial lesions since, similarly to what occurs in these patients, when they have to choose something that brings an immediate reward they tend to ignore the future consequences, at the risk of incurring a loss of reputation, job, home or family. Recent studies have indicated that impairment in decision-making may stand at the core of the problem of substance abuse [2].

In this chapter we will focus on the explanation of an important percentage of subjects with chronic substance use who present abnormalities in a prefrontal cortex (PFC) structure, the ventromedial prefrontal cortex (VMPFC), which turns out to be key in decision-making and, more specifically, in long-term prediction outcomes of a give action.

II. Origin, Anatomy and Function of the Prefrontal Cortex

Ontogeny recapitulates phylogeny. It is a basic principle in neuroanatomy, and the PFC is not an exception. In accordance to this principle, phylogenetically older brain areas mature earlier than newer ones. The PFC, the most recent brain region from an evolutionary point of view, supports this principle given that it is also the last region to reach maturity over the individual development.

Phylogeny

The PFC is part of the neocortex, also called isocortex or neopallium. This brain region evolves from two older structures: the archicortical region, originated in the hippocampus; and the paleocortical region, which emerged from the olfactory cortex [3].

The neocortex constitutes the 90% of all the cerebral cortex and, as its *neo* prefix indicates, this is the newest part of the cortex. This *young* region of the brain appears to be a hallmark of mammals, because its cytoarchitectural organization in 6 layers is not present in any other animal [4]. Similarly, due to disproportionate growth that PFC has undergone over the evolution, the PFC size constitutes a hallmark of the humans [5]. Thus, while the PFC constitutes

3.5% of the total cortex in the cat, 12.5% in the dog or 17% in the chimpanzee, the PFC in the human reaches 29% of the cortical surface [6].

Ontogeny

The general maturational pattern along the brain is such that, those regions involved in primary functions, such as motor or sensory areas, develop earlier; whereas the higher-order association areas, which integrate those more basic functions, develop later and only after the lower-order sensorimotor regions have matured [7]. The PFC constitutes the highest level of this hierarchy and, as mentioned above, it is the last region to reach maturity throughout individual development.

There are two processes of change in the development of the CPF that have been revealed as fundamental. The first of them has to do with the synaptic density, i.e., the number of synapses per unit volume of brain tissue. Early in postnatal development, the synaptic density increase due to the birth of new synapses (synaptogenesis). The number of synapses reaches it maximum at age 1-2 years and is about 50% above the adult levels [8]. Due to this resulting overproduction state, the synaptic proliferation process is followed by a period of synaptic pruning, which involve the elimination of infrequently used connections and the strengthening of frequently used ones. Unlike in sensory brain regions, where synaptic pruning and proliferation occurs relatively early during development, in the PFC an increase of synapses takes place at the onset of puberty [9]. This increasing is followed by pruning and strengthening of connections during adolescence, which results in a significant decrease in synaptic density (and, therefore, in gray matter) along this period [10]. This refinement synaptic process appears to be related to an improvement in neural networks functioning and, consequently, with increased neuronal efficiency [11-14].

The second major process involving PFC maturation is the myelination. Whereas sensory and motor areas become fully myelinated during the first years of life, the myelin sheaths generation in the PFC continues beyond adolescence [15]. As a consequence of myelination of connecting fibers in the PFC, an increase in speed of information processing takes place in this region throughout childhood and adolescence.

Since both myelination and synaptic reorganization processes entail a more efficient neural functioning, it is not surprising that development and organization of the PFC observed throughout childhood and adolescence lead to an improvement in cognitive functions support in part by this region such as attention, working memory, and inhibitory control [16].

Anatomy and Function

The PFC constitutes the association cortex of the frontal lobe. In human, it comprises areas 8-13, 32, and 44-47 according to the cytoarchitectonic map of Brodmann [3, 17]. The three major anatomical regions of the PFC are lateral, medial and ventral or orbital (see Figure 1). While the ventral and medial regions have been involved in emotional behavior, lateral region has been associated with spatial and conceptual reasoning processes [18]. Functionally, a gross but generally accepted division of the PFC is as follows: the dorsolateral prefrontal cortex (DLPFC), which would be involve in higher-order cognitive functions ("cold" processes), and the ventromedial prefrontal cortex (VMPFC), which would be related with affective/emotional functions ("hot" processes) [19].

Regarding the VMPFC, it is a wide region which includes both the gyrus rectus and mesial half of orbital gyri, as well as the inferior half of the medial prefrontal surface, from its most caudal aspect to the most rostral in the frontal pole [2]. Areas included in this region would be 10-13, 25, 32 and 47 of Brodmann (see Figure 2). The VMPFC is intimately connected with limbic structures involved in emotional processing as amygdala and hypothalamus [20]. The demonstrated involvement of VMPFC in inhibition, emotion and reward processing suggest a role in behavioral self-regulation and, therefore, in those disorders related with behavioral control such as obsessive compulsive disorder, antisocial personality or oppositional defiant disorder [21-23], as well as addiction or substance use disorders [24-26]. However, before addressing the relationship between the VMPFC and addictive behaviors, we will try to provide an updated approach of what is understood by addiction in accordance to different perspectives.

III. Addiction

The latest versions of the DSM defined substance dependence as a group of cognitive, behavioral, and physiological symptoms that indicate the loss of control over the use of a substance and that the person continues to use despite having problems related with the consumption. Moreover, if the substance is administered repeatedly, it can induce tolerance and withdrawal. That is, the continued use of the substance generates in the subject the need to continue using, which takes precedence over their interests and hobbies and generates, as a consequence, a progressive decline in the ability to control over consumption while it starts to change in the opinions, attitudes, and motivations related to the substance[27]. Thus, the subject becomes addicted (in a physiological level) and adept (in a psychological level), anticipating only the benefits and positive effects of the consumption.

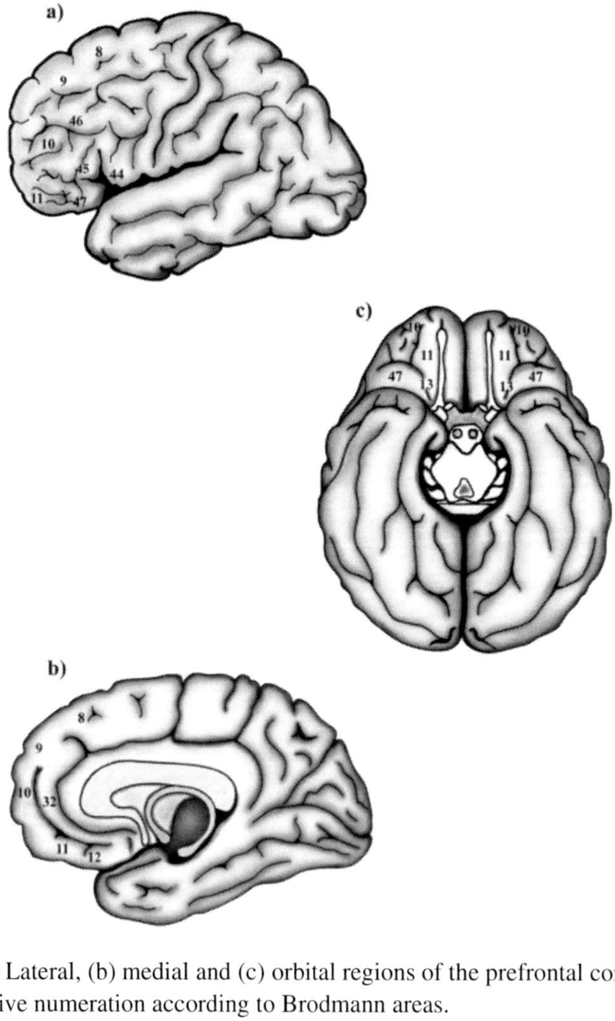

Figure 1. (a) Lateral, (b) medial and (c) orbital regions of the prefrontal cortex and their respective numeration according to Brodmann areas.

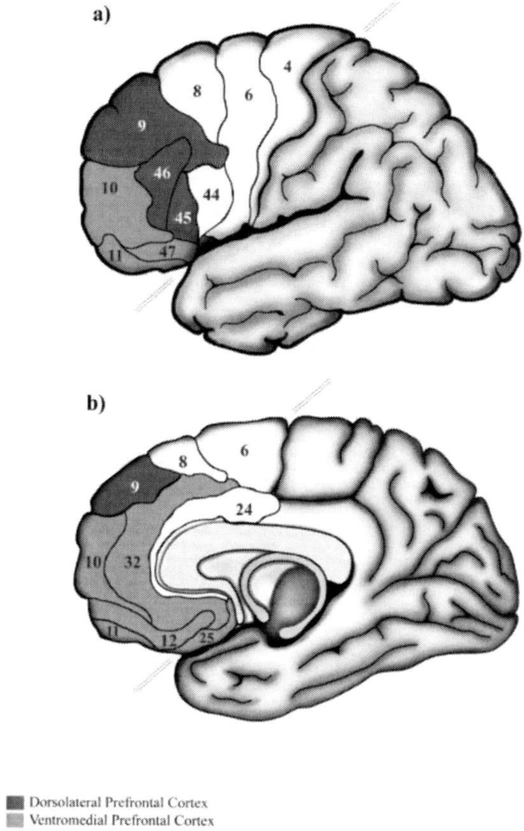

Figure 2. (a) Lateral and (b) medial view of the Brodmann areas of dorsolateral and ventromedial prefrontal cortex.

From a biological perspective, substance dependence may be understood as a dysfunction of the central nervous system related to mesencephalic brain structures, and cortical and limbic brain circuits involved in motivation and behavior [28-29]. We now know that chronic consumption of alcohol and other drugs produces neurobiological changes in different brain regions. These changes may induce motivational, emotional, decisional and cognitive changes as a result of compensatory biological responses to the pharmacological chronic effect of dugs in an attempt to reach the homeostasis again [30]. On the other hand, chronic use can leave an important mark on emotional memory, reshaping neural connections and pathways and producing long-lasting changes in brain functioning and leaving the individual more vulnerable to restart the consumption after quitting [29].

Besides the different approaches in the definition of *addiction* there are also controversies when explaining their acquisition and maintenance. In the 50s it was thought that drug use was maintained by negative reinforcement, for example, to cope with withdrawal symptoms or even to decrease negative internal states such as anxiety, stress, phobias, dysphoria or depression [30]. However, in the decade of the 60s laboratory findings showed that the behavior of drug administration was maintained in the absence of withdrawal, so that there was a conceptual change understanding that the addictive behavior would be explained by a process of positive reinforcement [31].

These changes in the conceptualization of the nature of addiction were reflected in the different editions of the DSM and ICD. Until de 80s addictions were included in personality disorders and it was the ICD-9 (1977), before DSM-III (1980), the first in grouping addictive disorders within a specific chapter which distinguished between dependence and abuse on alcohol or other drugs. This approach has been effective in the past 20 years along different editions and revisions and current proposals for DSM-V suggest that the diagnostic category could be called "Addiction and Related Disorders" which would include disordered gambling that has been encompassed until now within "Impulse Control Disorders". They will also dissappear the diagnoses of abuse and dependence being grouped into a single diagnosis of substance use disorder [32].

IV. Conceptualization of Addictions

Personality

Among individual factors that stand out in the explanation of the onset and maintenance of substance use are personality traits such as a high impulsivity and sensation seeking. Impulsivity is a personality trait that has classically been associated with addiction and with an early age of first consumption [33-37]. Within impulsivity we can distinguish: (1) a dimension that would be more related to the onset of the consumption due to difficulties to delay the reward and the need to obtain an immediate reinforcement; and (2) the rash impulsiveness, that would be involve in the maintenance of the consumption [33-34] and that is characterized by a rapid, spontaneous and even reckless response [38]. This last dimension of impulsivity is more related to the presence of comorbid psychopathology which may underlie a deficit in the frontal lobes [33, 38].

Sensation seeking is another personality trait that is defined as the need for new experiences and sensations, complex and varied, along with the willingness to take physical and social risks and it has been typically associated to drug use [39]. Regarding the relationship between sensation seeking, impulsivity and drug use, Belin and colleagues (2008) [40] suggested that sensation-seeking determines whether or not start using drugs, whilst impulsivity would be the emergence of abuse and dependence problems.

Rewarding Effect

From a behavioral point of view, the use of a psychoactive substance is regulated by its immediate consequences. Once the person consumes a drug, almost immediately, a pleasant effect occurs on the corresponding brain area [41]. The repetition of this behavior over time and across different situations will be generated widely in different situations becoming a well-established and durable habit.

In the initial stages of consumption, usually prevails a positive reinforcing effect, although some people with mental disorders or severe pain states can obtain powerful reinforcing effects due to unpleasant symptom relief. However, when the process is in advanced stages, positive reinforcing effects are less common but increasingly dominated by negative reinforcing effects of withdrawal relief [42].

Although the reinforcing effects of the substance are critical for learning the self-administration behavior, once the condicitining to internal and external stimuli has been consolidated, these conditioned stimuli may act as the signal to start the automated consumer behaviors without the need of mediation of cognitive processes of reflection, analysis, planning and behavioral inhibition, generated in the prefrontal cortex. That is, the conditioned stimuli can trigger conditioned responses of search and consumption that are beyond the volunteer control of the individual [41].

Drug Use as a Coping Strategy

There are many drugs that can improve the emotional state of the individual, which makes easier the subsequent process of abuse or dependence. The person suffering from unpleasant emotional states as anxiety, insomnia, phobias, worry, guilt, depression or insecurity perceive that substance use can help them to feel better and it seems to act as a relief of negative emotional states that can be very unpleasant or aversive [42]. However, these persons do not usually consider the subsequent rebound effect that occurs when the pharmacological effect ends. At this moment, symptoms reoccur with a greater intensity than the person felt before consumption. Nevertheless, it happens hours or days after and what remains strongly associated is the effect of immediate relief [30].

Biological Predisposition

Currently, it is known that some people are more prone to drug use than others. Biological predisposition does not imply causation, however, if the predisposed person tries a psychoactive substance this increases the risk in the continuation of the consumption, both by the biological processes of the substance and its reinforcement effects of the consumption [28, 43].

On the other hand, it has been commonly stated that when a subject presents a dependence on one or more substances this is because of clinical manifestations of a dysfunction on brain circuits involved in memory, learning, conditioning and inhibition of inappropriate responses. The chronic use of alcohol and other drugs produces motivational, emotional, decision-making, and other cognitive changes as a result of compensatory biological responses to the pharmacologic effect of these substances, in an attempt to establish new homeostatic balance. Moreover, poor performance of the VMPFC, which can occur in subjects with depression or conduct disorder, could manifest behaviorally as poor impulse control, an impaired ability to inhibit responses inappropriate and a low level of self-control behavior [2]. This could also explain the high propensity of adolescents to act impulsively and to ignore the potential negative consequences of their behavior, factors that increase the risk of substance abuse in this stage of life. The reason might be in the fact that those circuits involved in the regulation of emotions, reasoning ability and control of inappropriate responses are still immature during this period [44, 45].

In addition, all this plays an especially important role in relapse after the person quits. The ability to resist the urges for the consumption may depend on the ability to inhibit inappropriate responses. A dysfunction on regions that support these abilities, as the VMPFC, may involve a "disinhibition of inappropriate responses" of search and use of the substance [2].

Brain Reward Circuitry

The brain reward circuit is a primitive system, fundamental for the survival of both the individual and the species. On this system depend pleasure activities such as feeding or reproduction and it includes structures such as the ventral tegmental area, nucleus accumbens, and amygdala.

When primary reinforcing stimuli (those that are crucial for the survival and that play a critical role in motivational learning) is presented, dopamine neurons exhibit a phasic activation. This phasic activation produced by primary reinforcers (water, food, sexual behavior) also occurs with alcohol and other drugs because they produce an effect of dopamine release in the nucleus accumbens [46]. While primary reinforcers usually develop a fast tolerance or habituation, when it comes to psychoactive substances the behavior is different as the appetitive stimuli for these substances continue to act as dopamine triggers. Thus, unlike the "saciety" that comes after a consummatory behavior related to natural reinforces, drug appetitive or incentive effects can induce a desire to increase the consumption [29, 47]. Therefore, the drugs pervert the pleasure circuit that originally serves to facilitate to learn and to maintain the approach and consummatory behaviors, which are essential to the adaptation and the survival. What happens in the case of drugs is that the subject learns and tends to use them and at the same time keeps in his/her memory contextual stimuli that can serve later to trigger the consumption. This means that the last aim of the reward system is to perpetuate behaviors that give pleasure to the subject, and since substance use implies an increase of dopamine (the core neurotransmitter of this circuit), directly or indirectly, the hedonic effect is amplified. This feeling of pleasure is what makes the subject to consume again [46]. Therefore, the more intense the reinforcing effects of a substance, the most persistent are going to be the memories associated to it and bigger the necessity or *craving* (wanting) to experience them again.

In synthesis, both alcohol or other drugs activate the brain reward circuitry that is biologically related to survival, generating states of *need* for drugs that can be experienced subjectively as a need for survival and as a first priority for the addict subject.

Based on all the above, we can state that addictions cannot be explained only by genctic vulnerability factors, as in the step from one punctual use and a dependence are involved biological, psychological, and social factors as personality, educational environment, availability and accessibility of the substance, participation in different activities and healthy groups, negative reinforcers, etc. In some cases will prevail biological factors, in others the psychological, the social in others and a combination of all of them in others. This will influence in the onset, the maintenance and the escalation towards the consumption, and also for the abandonment of the drug. Related to this, it must be borne in mind that drugs of abuse have the potential to alter the structure and functioning brain of the brain as well as the way in which individuals learn and behave when they ingest them. The hypothesis that we will see next gives an explanation of how these anomalies in the structure and brain functioning may determine the behavior oriented to drugs.

V. The Somatic Marker Model

Among all the different conceptualizations of addiction that we have seen so far, in neuronscience it has drawn much of the attention a hypothesis that describes the addictive behavior as a disability to make decisions. Such alteration would be the product of a series of anomalies or disruptions in the brain systems that underlie the ability to make decisions. Before addressing how these dysfunctions can take place and how these anomalies may affect compulsive drug use, it is necessary to establish the conceptual framework of the somatic marker model on which the bases for the explanation of the addictive behavior are underpinned.

The Somatic Marker Hypothesis

Imagine that you are on the dilemma of making a decision, for example, which dish to choose in an exotic restaurant, as can be a Thai restaurant. After browsing the restaurant menu and seeing the variety of dishes, you will probably (if you come from more occidental culinary traditions) discard immediately the options of eating monkey brains, dry lizard, or bee larvae. The reason for this is that when the result of a given future option appears in our mind (our own image eating bee larvae, for example), we experiment, although briefly, an unpleasant feeling in the bowels, in the body, i.e., a *somatic* state that determines or *mark* (the image of) the option that we are taking into account. In this case, the option of eating bee larvae causes a negative emotional state (a negative somatic marker) that leads to reject this choice. On the other hand, if we check that in the menu there is the *Khanon Djied* and we remind the pleasant aroma and the rich flavour that this dish had the last time we had it, it is likely that we select this option, because a somatic state has again marked (this time positively) one of the response options that we had.

This would constitute essentially the basis for the hypothesis of the somatic marker. A collection of body- and brain-related signals, that emerge during the process of pondering decisions, and that are linked to the immediate or future results of a particular response option. Within this scheme, when a negative signal juxtaposes to a particular result, the combination implies the reject of this option. In contrast, when what juxtaposes is a positive signal, this combination leads to choose this option [1, 48]. Of course, the mechanisms that determine a decision may be more complex and multiple signals with positive or negative valence could coexist. The "winner" signal, which decants the choice, seems to follow the principles of the natural selection: stronger signals prevail on weaker signals [49-50].

These somatic markers are a guide in the decision-making process, "bringing closer" the subjects to adaptive decisions for his/ her survival and "distancing them" of those actions that result maladaptive. A defect in the neural circuitry that underlies the emotional signals processing assigned to a certain choice would involve a *myopia for the future*, i.e., a disability to advance possible positive or negative consequences of certain actions. Under the umbrella of this interpretation, it is possible that people with a substance abuse disorder present a disability in these neural systems that leads them to an incorrect evaluation of the long-term consequences of their behavior and/or to overvalue the rewarding impact of drugs. We will see, before assessing this interpretation, which are the circuits implied in the emotional signals associated with a certain choice.

Somatic States and Their Neural Substrates

The somatic marker model proposes that emotions are a fundamental axis in the decision-making process. From a neurophysiological point of view, there are two neural circuits that are critical for this process; the *impulsive neural system*, in which the amygdala is the key structure, and the *reflective neural system*, in which is the VMPFC what plays a critical role [50]. Although both structures link exteroceptive sensory information to interoceptive information concerning somatic states, they play different roles since they are activated from different inductors.

The amygdala is a critical substrate in the neural system associated with triggering somatic states from *primary inducers*. These primary inducers are stimuli or entities that, unconditionally or through learning, can produce states that are pleasurable or aversive. Facing with a snake in the countryside or watching the “wriggle” on the grass (a stimulus predictive of a snake), an actual encounter of a drug by a drug user, or semantic information such as gaining or losing large amounts of money, are all of them primary inducers.

Of course, although the amygdala is the key structure in the impulsive neural system, this nucleus is not alone. The thalamus (covertly or non-consciously) and the primary sensory and higher-order association cortices (overtly or consciously) are involved in processing the features of primary inducers. Hypothalamus, nucleus accumbens, basal forebrain or periaqueductal gray substance, are some of the effector structures engaged in evoke a somatic state. Inside this system, the role of the amygdala is to connect the information from thalamus and/or primary and higher-order association cortices with the hypothalamus and the autonomic nuclei in brain stem (the effector structures). Once somatic states are induced, signals from these somatic states are transmitted to the brain. If these signals reach the insula and surrounding somatosensory cortices they will be perceived as a *feeling*. Concurrently, the somatic states can also activate the motivational systems, such as anterior cingulated cortex, and the motor effector structures, such as striatum and supplementary motor area, associated with the decision to select or to reject a response (see Figure 3).

The VMPFC is a critical region inside the neural system necessary for the processing of *secondary inducers*. The secondary inducers are entities generated by “thoughts” or “memories” of the primary inducers. When these entities are brought to working memory they can trigger a somatic state. The imagination of winning an important amount of money, the recall of encountering a snake or having a drug experience, are all examples of secondary inducers.

The VMPFC couples 1) recalled or imagined events (secondary inducers) supported by higher-order association cortices important for memory, such as the DLPFC, to 2) the effector structures that induce the somatic states and to 3) the neural systems involved in the representation of the somatic states (the *feeling*), such as the insular and somatosensory cortices (see Figure 4).

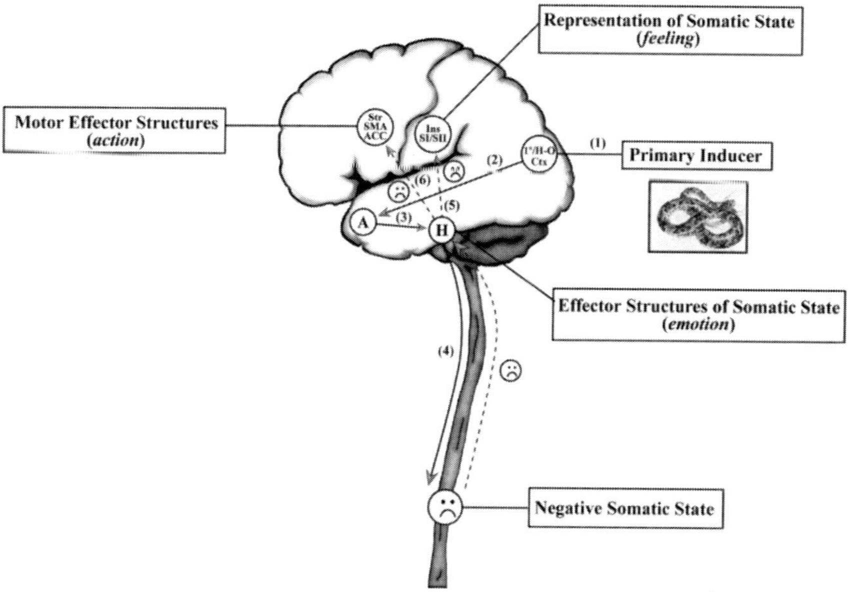

Figure 3. Schematic representation of neural circuitry of impulsive system. (1) Once a primary inducer (e.g., a snake) is processed by thalamus or primary sensory/higher-order association cortices (1°/H-O Ctx), (2) the information is relayed to amygdala (A). (3) This nucleus sends the information about the primary inducer to the effector structures, i.e., hypothalamus and autonomic nuclei of brainstem (H), (4) which are responsible for inducing the somatic state. Representations of this signal (e.g., the negative somatic state related to the image of a snake) can remain covert at the brain stem level, or (5) it can reach the insula (Ins) and the somatosensory cortex (SI /SII) and, consequently, to be perceived as a feeling. Concurrently, (6) the somatic states can also activate the motor effector structures –striatum (Str), supplementary motor area (SMA) and anterior cingulated cortex (ACC)- associated with the decision to select a response (e.g., escape from the snake).

The Role of VMPFC in Decision-Making

The knowledge of the role of the VMPFC in the processing of emotions and, consequently, in decision-making, comes from studies with patients who had lesions in this region. These subjects are characterized by a marked inability to take into account long-term consequences when making a decision. Despite they usually preserve normal intelligence and have similar performance than the normal population in a wide range of neuropsychological tasks, their ability to experience and to express emotions as well as their social behavior are significantly impaired. Often, VMPFC patients make decisions that entail loss of money, reputation, job or even home or family. Furthermore, they tend to deny or to not be aware that they have a problem in spite of the negative consequences of their behavior.

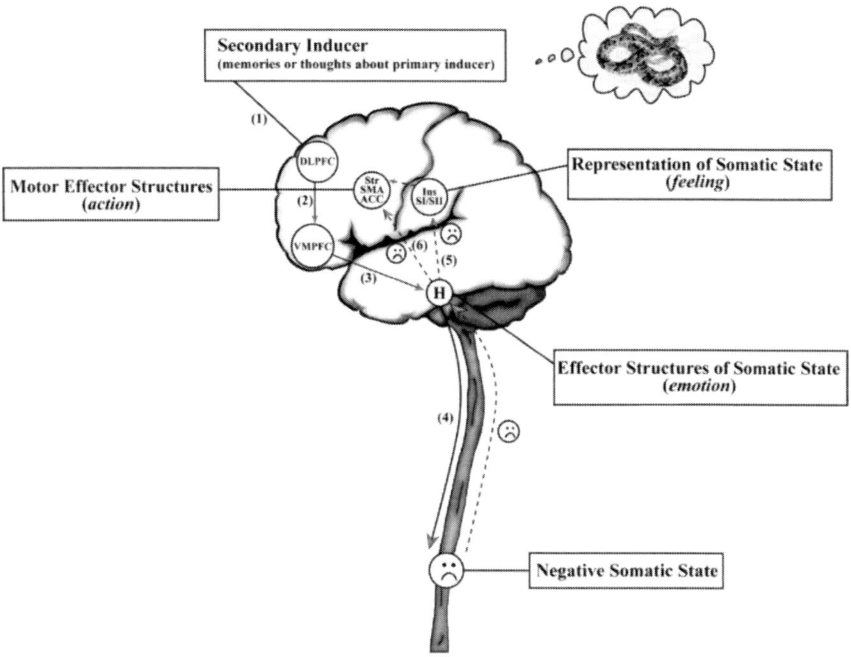

Figure 4. Schematic representation of the neural circuitry of reflective system. (1) Memories or thoughts about the primary inducers (e.g., the image of a snake) are brought to memory by higher-order association cortices, such as dorsolateral prefrontal cortex (DLPFC), which (2) send this information to ventromedial prefrontal cortex (VMPFC). (3) The VMPFC connects information about the secondary inducer (the image of a snake) with the effector structures that induce the somatic states – hypothalamus and autonomic nuclei of brainstem (H). (4) Once the somatic state is triggered, it can remain covert at the brain stem level, or (5) can reach the insula (Ins) and the somatosensory cortex (SI /SII) and, consequently, to be perceived as a feeling. (6) At the same time, the somatic states can also activate the motor effector structures – striatum (Str), the supplementary motor area (SMA) and the anterior cingulated cortex (ACC)- associated with the decision to select a response (e.g., escape from the snake).

With the aim of studying possible deficits in the decision-making process in VMPFC patients, the research group of Iowa University developed the *gambling task* [51]. This task simulates real-life situations since its execution involves potential rewards and punishments in conditions of uncertainty and risk. During the task the subjects have to choose between decks of cards that yield high gain in short-term but larger loss in long-term, and decks that yield lower gain in short-term but smaller loss in long-term. Two decks of cards are disadvantageous over the long-term (even though they bring higher immediate reward), while the other two decks are advantageous in the long-term (i.e., the long-term losses are smaller than the short-term gains, thus yielding a net profit). Healthy subjects tend to avoid the disadvantageous or "risky" decks (those with high immediate gains but larger future loss) and to pick the advantageous or "safe" decks (those with lower immediate gain but smaller future loss). In contrast, patients with VMPFC lesions tend to opt for choices that yield immediate gains but larger future loss, so before they finish the task they are "in the red". This decision-making deficit has been labeled as *myopia for the future* [52]. VMPFC patients are unable to use ongoing feedback to guide future responses, and therefore evaluate each decision in terms only of the immediate reward available. This performance profile is consistent with their real-life inability to make suitable decisions.

VI. Vetromedial Prefrontal Cortex, Addictive Behavior and *Myopia* for the Future

At the beginning of the century, Bechara et al. [53] proposed that substance dependent subjects were similar to patients with VMPFC lesions in two principal aspects: 1) they both tend to deny or to be not aware that they have a problem; and 2) when they are involved in situations in which they have to make a decision that implies immediate reward, at the risk of incurring future adverse results, they tend to choose the immediate reward and to ignore the future consequences.

Since then, several studies examining performance of substance dependent subjects in the gambling task have consistently shown significant impairments in their decision-making process [52, 54-58]. The difficulty to stop using the substance in these patients is attributed to a defect in the neural circuit that subserves to emotional response to drugs. More specifically, the conflict of taking or not a drug is resolve when somatic signals triggered by either the impulsive neural system or the reflective neural system prevail [59]. Under this interpretation, two types of dysfunctions in substance dependent individuals are possible:

(1) a hyperactivation of the amygdala (and therefore of the impulsive neural system), which magnify the rewarding impact of available incentives, and
(2) an hypoactivativation of the VMPFC (and therefore of the reflective neural system), which underestimates the future consequences of a particular action. Substance dependent subjects may have impaired one or both of these systems.

For a better understanding of the VMPFC dysfunctions in addiction, and based on the schematic model of somatic marker detailed in [52] a simplified representation about the decision-making process in this subtype of substance dependents subjects has been elaborated (see Figure 5). To see the profile of the other subtypes of substance dependent individuals, the authors refer the reader to the studies of Bechara and cols. [52, 54]

As can be observed in Figure 5a, after a primary inducer of reward, such as food (e.g., a chocolate cake), is processed via thalamus or primary/higher-order sensory areas, it reaches the amygdala. This nucleus relays the information of the primary inducer to hypothalamus and autonomic nuclei in brain stem, the effector structures that induce the somatic response (e.g., a pleasure somatic state related to the food).

On the other hand, the processing of the primary inducer can trigger, in turn, "thoughts" or "memories" (e.g., an image of ourselves with overweight) that are brought to awareness by higher-order association cortices (such as DLPFC). These secondary inducers are connected with the effector structures that induce the somatic states by means of the VMPFC. Under normal circumstances, there is a "neural competition" between the impulsive and the reflective systems or, in other words, between the negative and the positive markers. Once one of these signals (positive or negative) *wins* or prevails, the feeling concerning to the *winner* somatic state emerges. At the end of the process, the winner provides the substrate for biasing the decision to select a response through motivational systems, such as anterior cingulated cortex, and motor effector structures, such as striatum and supplementary motor area. In this case, the winner would be the negative somatic state associated with the overweight image, so the election of eating the chocolate cake is rejected.

In the case of substance dependent subjects with a dysfunction in the VMPFC (Figure 5b), the primary inducer would be a bottle of wine and the secondary inducer would be the thoughts about negative consequences concerning, for example, the hangover symptoms. In these subjects, although the negative image from higher-order cortices is generated (the hangover symptoms), VMPFC is not capable to induce a somatic response or it is too weak to *compete* with the signal induced from impulsive neural system. Thus, in the "neural competition" between the impulsive (amygdala) and the reflective (VMPFC) systems, the winner will be the impulsive neural system and, therefore, the positive somatic state associated with drinking a bottle of wine prevails.

Although this is a schematic view of the addictive behavior, this representation allows to explain, from a neurocognitive perspective, why substance dependent subjects with VMPFC dysfunction continue using drugs even when they experience physical, psychological and/or social problems. These individuals do not take into account the long-term consequences of their behavior and, consequently, they tend to choose the immediate reward at expense of severe negative future consequences. This is, in essence, what the term *myopia for the future* means.

Addiction and VMPFC: Scientific Evidences

There is a growing scientific evidence that suggest that a decision-making impairment linked to a dysfunctional VMPFC may be at the core of substances dependence. A common paradigm to examine the relationship between decision-making, VMPFC function, and addiction has been the gambling task. Several studies have shown that the performance on the gambling task is associated with activity in the VMPFC. As we discussed in the previous section, lesion studies have demonstrated that damage in the VMPFC impairs the performance on the gambling task [2]. Likewise, neuroimaging and electrophysiological studies have indicated that the VMPFC is active during the performance of this task [60-61]. These studies suggest that the gambling task is a valid instrument to assess the decision-making mediated by the VMPFC.

Regarding substance dependents subjects, studies have shown that chronic drug users such as alcohol, cannabis, cocaine, opioids, MDMA or methamphetamines have a poor performance in the gambling and other similar tasks [62-68]. An impairment in decision-making have also been reported in populations with a high risk for drug abuse, such as individuals without prior alcohol exposure but with higher family density of alcoholism [69-70], individuals with pathological gambling [71-72], as well as adolescents with a binge drinking pattern of alcohol consumption [73-75] or with externalizing behavior disorders [76-77].

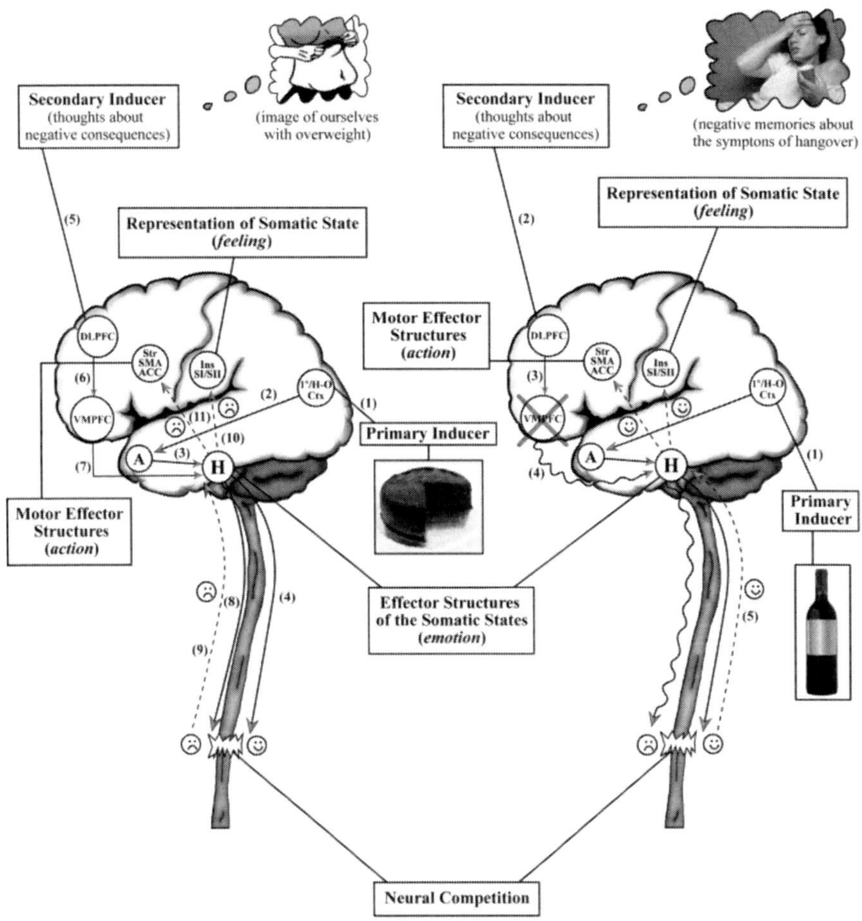

(a) (b)

Figure 5. (a) (1) A primary inducer of reward, such as food (e.g., a chocolate cake), is processed via thalamus or primary/higher-order sensory areas (1°/H-O Ctx). (2) The signal about this primary inducer reaches the amygdala. (3) This nucleus relay the information to the effector structures of somatic state –hypothalamus and autonomic nuclei of brainstem (H)-, which (4) induce the positive somatic state associated with the primary inducer. On the other hand, (5) dorsolateral prefrontal cortex (DLPFC) and other higher-order association cortices involved in memory processes can evoke "thoughts" or "memories" directly or indirectly related to the primary inducer (e.g., an image of ourselves with overweight) and (6) send this information to ventromedial prefrontal cortex (VMPFC). (7) The VMPFC couples the information about the secondary inducer (the image of ourselves with overweight) to the effector structures that induce the somatic states –hypothalamus and autonomic nuclei of brainstem (H). (8) After this somatic state is induced, under normal circumstances, there is a "neural competition" between the somatic state induced via ventromedial prefrontal cortex and the somatic state induced via amygdala. (9) Once one of these signals *wins* or prevails (e.g., the negative somatic state associated with the image of ourselves with overweight), (10) the feeling concerning to the *winner* somatic signal may emerge. At the same time, (11) this signal activates the motor effector systems –striatum (Str) and supplementary motor area (SMA) and anterior cingulated cortex (ACC)- providing the basis for selecting a response (e.g., refuse the chocolate cake).

(b) In substance dependents individuals (1) an "encounter" with a drug (e.g., a bottle of wine) can constitute a primary inducer. In the subtype of substance dependents subjects with a dysfunction in the VMPFC, (2) although the secondary inducer from higher-order cortices can be generated (e.g., the negative thought about the symptoms of hangover) and (3) their information sent to the VMPFC, (4) this structure is not capable to induce a somatic response or it is too weak to *compete* with the signal induced from the amygdala. Thus, in the "neural competition" between the impulsive (amygdala) and the reflective (VMPFC) neural systems, (5) the winner would be the impulsive neural system. Finally, the positive somatic state associated with drinking a bottle of wine prevails and, ultimately, the decision will be in relation with such somatic state (e.g., drinking the bottle of wine).

Similarly, structural brain impairments involving VMPFC and other regions related to somatic states activation and decision-making processes have been shown in substance dependent individuals. In that sense, a significant decrease in grey matter volume throughout these brain regions have been repeatedly observed in chronic drug users, which has been associated with disadvantages in decision-making [78-82]. Substance dependent individuals also showed abnormalities in white matter microstructure of VMPFC [83-86], which could reflect disruptions in connectivity between VMPFC and other regions involved in decision-making.

Studies with functional Magnetic Resonance Imaging (fMRI) have also showed significant impairments in substance dependent subjects in neural regions that are critical for the somatic marker circuitry. Regarding VMPFC, neuroimaging studies have revealed a decreased activation in this region during decision-making processes in chronic drug users compared to healthy subjects [87-88]. This VMPFC hypoactivity appears to lead to a difficulty in the prediction of the long-term consequences. Likewise, a dysfunction in VMPFC are also involved in aspects of greater relevance for prevention and treatment of addictive behaviors, such as *craving* [89-91] and risk of relapse [92-94].

Of course, the VMPFC is not the only region of PFC that seems to be related to drug use and abuse. Integrity of DLPFC is also necessary for a correct functioning of the reflective system. In that sense, damage in DLPFC can indirectly affect to VMPFC functioning, and thus alter the normal operation of the reflective system. Several studies have shown that working memory disruptions can lead to poor decision-making in substance dependent subjects [95-97].

Together, these findings reinforce the applicability of somatic marker model to the study of addictive behavior. According to this perspective, addiction is seen as a condition in which subjects are unable to choose according to future outcomes. The VMPFC, a critical region for making decisions that are advantageous in the long-term, have consistently shown to be impaired in substance dependent individuals. Thus, VMPFC dysfunction appears to be involved in the inability of some chronic drug users to stop using drugs in spite of their negative consequences.

VII. Implications for the Treatment

The somatic marker hypothesis points out that the subjects with substance dependence have difficulties when making a decision. This may have important consequences when trying to quit and to maintain abstinence.

Accordingly, the somatic marker model of addiction has several implications for the clinical treatment. Taking into account that emotions play a fundamental role in the decision-making process, treatments that usually are conducted with drug addicted individuals should focus, in addition to the cognitive aspects –which have attracted much of the attention-, on the emotional dimension. Likewise, pharmacological treatments alone might not be the best strategy in the way to rehabilitation since the person also needs to *re-learn* how to think and behave in situations related to drugs while treated with medications. Reversal of the possible chemical deficiency would not be enough for improving the decision-making process [59]. Drug treatment along with a *re-learning* therapy could be an effective strategy to restore the decision-making ability in subjects with substance abuse. Therapies that have impact on the ability of individuals to plan their daily activities, to make everyday decisions or to be conscious about their drug-related problems are examples of possible ways to re-establish the ability to make advantageous choices [98].

In the same way, the counselling sessions themselves may activate frontal-cortical executive functions increasing frontal lobe function, thus reducing impulsivity and preventing relapse [26]. An effective therapy in substance dependents subjects should increase individual motivation to make him or her going through the different stages of change: contemplation, preparation, action and maintenance; as all of them depend on executive function and, therefore, on the PFC [26, 99].

Finally, the factors that regulate the persistence of dependence as well as motivation to control or to avoid addictive behaviors are relaying on the decisional balance between reflective and impulsive systems [26]. As we have seen above, substance dependent subjects with an unbalance in this neural systems (e.g., hypoactivity in the reflective system) will probably show deficits in the ability to control their addictive behavior, since it is the immediate reward which guides their acts (the impulsive system) and there is not an evaluation of the future consequences of such acts. Once more, treatments aimed to reduce the rewarding effect of drugs and to try to develop the ability to assess the future consequences, are important strategies when restoring the decision-making ability in the addicted individual.

CONCLUSION

Addiction is a very complex entity whose conceptualization has change over the years. In the last decade, a perspective that has drawn much of the attention in neuroscience is the somatic marker hypothesis, which describes the addictive behavior as a disability to make decisions. Following this perspective, growing scientific evidence has related the poor decision-making ability frequently observed in addiction to disruptions in functioning of a distributed neural network critical for the processing of emotion. Inside this network, the VMPFC has a central role in the decision-making process, especially in the evaluation of positive or negative consequences of a given action. Under this interpretation, substance dependents subjects with a dysfunction in the VMPFC appear to be unable to take into account the long-term consequences of continued drug use and, consequently, they tend to choose the immediate reward (the drug consumption) at expense of severe negative future consequences.

The main contribution of this model is that it provides an explanation of the inability in drug addicted individuals for choosing short-term outcomes rather than long-term ones through a systems-level neuroanatomical and cognitive framework [2]. Future studies should investigate the relationship between structure abnormalities and behavioral domains associated with decision-making in drug dependent individuals. Longitudinal studies are also needed to determine if brain alterations in decision-making and impulse control are a consequence or if they precede drug abuse.

Acknowledgments

The authors thank the illustrator Carlos Rodríguez Brea for having designed the images. The chapter was supported by the FPU program (AP2008-03433) of the Spanish *Ministerio de Educación* and by the *Plan Galego de Investigación, Innovación e Crecemento 2011-2015 (Plan I2C)* of Xunta de Galicia.

References

[1] Damasio, A.R. (1994). *Descartes' Error: Emotion, Reason, and the Human Brain.* Grosset/Putnam, New York.

[2] Bechara, A., Damasio, H. & Damasio, A. R. (2000). Emotion, decision making and the orbitofrontal cortex. *Cereb Cortex*, *10*, 295-307.

[3] Pandya, D. N. & Yeterian, E. H. (1996). Comparison of prefrontal architecture and connections. *Philos Trans R Soc Lond B Biol Sci*, *351*, 1423-32.

[4] Rakic, P. (2009). Evolution of the neocortex: a perspective from developmental biology. *Nat Rev Neurosci*, *10*, 724-35.

[5] Jerison, H. J. (1994). Evolution of the brain. In: Zaidel, DW, editor. Neuropsicolgia (Handbook of perception and cognition). San Diego, CA, US: Academic Press, 53-82.

[6] Fuster, J. M. (2008). The Prefrontal Cortex. Fourth Edition. Boston: Academic Press.

[7] Gogtay, N., Giedd, J. N., Lusk, L., Hayashi, K. M., Greenstein, D., Vaituzis, A. C. & Nugent, T. F. 3rd, Herman, D. H., Clasen, L. S., Toga, A. W., Rapoport, J. L. & Thompson, P. M. (2004). Dynamic mapping of

human cortical development during childhood through early adulthood. *Proc Natl Acad Sci USA*, *101*, 8174-9.

[8] Huttenlocher, P. R. (1979). Synaptic density in human frontal cortex - developmental changes and effects of aging. *Brain Res*, *163*,195-205.

[9] Giedd, J. N., Blumenthal, J., Jeffries, N. O., Castellanos, F. X., Liu, H., Zijdenbos, A., Paus, T., Evans, A. C. & Rapoport, J. L. (1999). Brain development during childhood and adolescence: a longitudinal MRI study. *Nat Neurosci*, *2*, 861-3.

[10] Sowell, E. R., Thompson, P. M., Tessner, K. D. & Toga, A. W. (2001). Mapping continued brain growth and gray matter density reduction in dorsal frontal cortex: Inverse relationships during postadolescent brain maturation. *J Neurosci*, *21*, 8819-29.

[11] Casey, B. J., Giedd, J. N. & Thomas, K. M. (2000). Structural and functional brain development and its relation to cognitive development. *Biol Psychol*, *54*, 241-57.

[12] Casey, B. J., Tottenham, N., Liston, C. & Durston, S. (2005). Imaging the developing brain: what have we learned about cognitive development? *Trends Cogn Sci*, *9*, 104-10.

[13] Hua, J. Y. & Smith, S. J. (2004). Neural activity and the dynamics of central nervous system development. *Nat Neurosci*, *7*, 327–32.

[14] de Graaf-Peters, V. B. & Hadders-Algra, M. (2006). Ontogeny of the human central nervous system: what is happening when? *Early Hum Dev*, *82*, 257–66.

[15] Lebel, C. & Beaulieu, C. (2011). Longitudinal development of human brain wiring continues from childhood into adulthood. *J Neurosci*, *31*, 10937-47

[16] Luna, B., Garver, K. E., Urban, T. A., Lazar, N. A., Sweeney, J. A. (2004). Maturation of cognitive processes from late childhood to adulthood. *Child Dev*, *75*, 1357-72.

[17] Fuster, J. M. (2001). The prefrontal cortex--an update: time is of the essence. *Neuron*, *30*, 319-33.

[18] Stuss, D. T. & Levine, B. (2002). Adult clinical neuropsychology: lessons from studies of the frontal lobes. *Annu Rev Psychol*, *53*, 401-33.

[19] Goldstein, R. Z. & Volkow, N. D. (2011). Dysfunction of the prefrontal cortex in addiction: neuroimaging findings and clinical implications. *Nat Rev Neurosci*, *12*, 652-69.

[20] Damasio, A. R. (1995). On some functions of the human prefrontal cortex. *Ann N Y Acad Sci*, *769*, 241-51.

[21] Everitt, B. J. & Robbins, T. W. (2005). Neural systems of reinforcement for drug addiction: from actions to habits to compulsion. *Nat Neurosci*, *8*, 1481-9.

[22] Mazas, C. A., Finn, P. R; Steinmetz, J. E. (2000). Decision-making biases, antisocial personality, and early-onset alcoholism. *Alcohol Clin Exp Res*, *24*, 1036-40.

[23] Finger, E. C., Marsh, A. A., Mitchell, D. G., Reid, M. E., Sims, C., Budhani, S., Kosson, D. S., Chen, G., Towbin, K. E., Leibenluft, E., Pine, D. S., Blair, J. R. (2008). Abnormal ventromedial prefrontal cortex function in children with psychopathic traits during reversal learning. *Arch Gen Psychiatry*, *65*, 586-94.

[24] Volkow, N. D., Fowler, J. S. (2000). Addiction, a disease of compulsion and drive: involvement of the orbitofrontal cortex. *Cereb Cortex*, *10*, 318-25.

[25] Koob, G. F., Ahmed, S. H., Boutrel, B., Chen, S. A., Kenny, P. J., Markou, A., O'Dell, L. E., Parsons, L. H. & Sanna, P. P. (2004). Neurobiological mechanisms in the transition from drug use to drug dependence. *Neurosci Biobehav Rev*, *27*, 739-49.

[26] Crews, F. T. & Boettiger, C. A. (2009). Impulsivity, frontal lobes and risk for addiction. *Pharmacol Biochem Behav*, *93*, 237-47.

[27] American Psychiatric Association. (2000). Diagnostic and statistical manual for mental disorders, 4th ed., revised text. Washington, DC: American Psychiatric Association.

[28] Leshner, A. I. (1997). Addiction is a brain disease, and it matters. *Science*, *278*, 45-7.

[29] Kalivas, P. W. & Volkow, N. D. (2005). The neural basis of addiction: a pathology of motivation and choice. *Am J Psychiatry*, *162*, 1403-13.

[30] Guardia, S. J., Surkov, S. & Cardús, M. (2010). Neurobiología de la Adicción. In: Pereiro, C, editor. Manual de Adicciones para médicos especialistas en formación. Socidrogalcohol. *Barcelona*, 37-130.

[31] Stolerman, I. (1992). Drugs of abuse: behavioral principles, methods and terms. *Trends Pharmacol Sci*, *13*, 170-6.

[32] O'Brien, C. (2010). Addiction and dependence in DSM-V. *Addiction*, *106*, 866-7.

[33] Dawe, S., Gullo, M. J. & Loxton, N. J. (2004). Reward drive and rash impulsiveness as dimensions of impulsivity: implications for substance misuse. *Addictive Behaviors*, *29*, 1389-405.

[34] Forcada, R., Pardo, N. & Bondía, B. (2006). Impulsividad en dependientes de cocaína que abandonan el consumo. *Adicciones*, *18*, 111-8.

[35] Tarter, R. E., Kirisci, L., Mezzich, A., Cornelius, J. R., Pajer, K., Vanyukov, M. & Clark, D. (2003). Neurobehavioral disinhibition in childhood predicts early age at onset of substance use disorder. *American Journal of Psychiatry*, *160*, 1078-85.

[36] Verdejo-García, A., Lawrence, A. J. & Clark, L. (2008). Impulsivity as a vulnerability marker for substance-use disorders: review of findings from high-risk research, problem gamblers and genetic associatio studies. *Neuroscience and Behavioral Reviews*, *32*, 777-810.

[37] Von Diemen, L., García, D., Costa, S., Maciel, C. & Pechansky, F. (2008). Impulsivity, age of first alcohol use and substance use disorders among male adolescents: a population based case-control study. *Addiction*, *103*, 1198-205.

[38] Dawe, S. & Loxton, N. J. (2004). The role of impulsivity in the development of substance use and eating disorders. *Neuroscience and Biobehavioral Reviews*, *28*, 343-51.

[39] Zuckerman, M. (1979). Sensation seeking: Beyond the optimal level of arousal. Hillsdale, NJ: Erlbaum.

[40] Belin, D., Mar, A. C., Dalley, J. W., Robbins, T. W. & Everitt, B. J. (2008). High impulsivity predicts the switch to compulsive cocaine-taking. *Science*, *320*, 1352-5.

[41] Hyman, S. E. & Malenka, R. C. (2001). Addiction and the brain: the neurobiology of comupulsion and its persistence. *Nat Rev Neurosci*, *2*, 695-703

[42] Eissenberg, T. (2004). Measuring the emergence of tobacco dependence: the contribution of negative reinforcement models. *Addiction*, *99*, 5-29.

[43] Becoña, E. (2002). *Bases científicas de la prevención de las drogodependencias.* Madrid: Delegación del Gobierno para el Plan Nacional sobre Drogas.

[44] Luna, B. & Sweeney, J. A. (2004). The emergence of collaborative brain function: FMRI studies of the development of response inhibition. *Ann New York Acad Sci*, *1021*, 296-309.

[45] Chambers, R. A., Taylor, J. R. & Potenza, M. N. (2003). Developmental neurocircuitry of motivation in adolescence: a critical period of addiction vulnerability. *American Journal of Psychiatry*, *160*, 1041-52.

[46] Tirapu, J., Landa, N. & Lorea, I. (2004). Cerebro y adicción. Una guía comprensiva. Navarra: Gobierno de Navarra Departamento de Salud.

[47] Hyman, S. E., Malenka, R. C. & Nestler, E. J. (2006). Neural mechanisms of addiction: the role of reward-related learning and memory. *Annu Rev Neurosci*, *29*, 565-98.

[48] Damasio, A. R. (1996). The somatic marker hypothesis and the possible functions of the prefrontal cortex. *Philos Trans R Soc Lond B Biol Sci*, *351*, 1413-20.

[49] Bechara, A. & Damasio, A. R. (2005). The somatic marker hypothesis: a neural theory of economic decision. Games Econ. *Behav*. *52*, 336–72.

[50] Bechara, A. (2005). Decision making, impulse control and loss of willpower to resist drugs: a neurocognitive perspective. *Nat Neurosci*, *8*, 1458-63.

[51] Bechara, A., Damasio, A. R., Damasio, H. & Anderson, S. W. (1994). Insensitivity to future consequences following damage to human prefrontal cortex. *Cognition*, *50*, 7-15.

[52] Bechara, A., Dolan, S. & Hindes, A. (2002). Decision-making and addiction (part II): myopia for the future or hypersensitivity to reward? *Neuropsychologia*, *40*, 1690-705.

[53] Bechara, A., Dolan, S., Denburg, N., Hindes, A., Anderson, S. W. & Nathan, P. E. (2001). Decision-making deficits, linked to a dysfunctional ventromedial prefrontal cortex, revealed in alcohol and stimulant abusers. *Neuropsychologia*, *39*, 376-89.

[54] Bechara, A. & Damasio, H. (2002). Decision-making and addiction (part I): impaired activation of somatic states in substance dependent individuals when pondering decisions with negative future consequences. *Neuropsychologia*, *40*, 1675-89.

[55] Hanson, K. L., Luciana, M. & Sullwold, K. (2008). Reward-related decision-making deficits and elevated impulsivity among MDMA and other drug users. *Drug Alcohol Depend*, *96*, 99-110.

[56] Quednow, B. B., Kuhn, K. U., Hoppe, C., Westheide, J., Maier, W., Daum, I. & Wagner, M. (2007). Elevated impulsivity and impaired decision-making cognition in heavy users of MDMA ("Ecstasy"). *Psychopharmacology (Berl)*, *189*, 517-30.

[57] Stout, J. C., Busemeyer, J. R., Lin, A., Grant, S. J. & Bonson, K. R. (2004). Cognitive modeling analysis of decision-making processes in cocaine abusers. *Psychol Bull Rev*, *4*, 742–7.

[58] Verdejo-García, A. & Pérez-García, M. (2007). Profile of executive deficits in cocaine and heroin polysubstance users: common and differential effects on separate executive components. *Psychopharmacology (Berl)*, *190*, 517-30.

[59] Verdejo-Garcia, A. & Bechara, A. (2009). A somatic marker theory of addiction. *Neuropharmacology*, *56*, Suppl 1, 48-62.

[60] Adolphs, R., Bechara, A., Kaufman, O., Kawasaki, H., Bakken, H., Damasio, H., Granner, M. & Howard III, M. (2000). Single-unit responses in human orbitofrontal cortex: Decision-making on a gambling task. Seventh Ann. Meeting Cog. Neurosci. Soc., MIT Press, San Francisco.

[61] Ernst, M., Bolla, K., Mouratidis, M., Contoreggi, C., Matochik, J. A., Kurian, V., Cadet, J., Kimes, A. S. & London, E. D. (2002). Decision-

making in a risk-taking task: a PET study. *Neuropsychopharmacology, 26*, 682–691.

[62] Rogers, R. D., Everitt, B. J., Baldacchino, A., Blackshaw, A. J., Swainson, R., Wynne, K., Baker, N. B., Hunter, J., Carthy, T., Booker, E., London, M., Deakin, J. F., Sahakian, B. J. & Robbins, T. W. (1999). Dissociable deficits in the decision-making cognition of chronic amphetamine abusers, opiate abusers, patients with focal damage to prefrontal cortex, and tryptophan-depleted normal volunteers: evidence for monoaminergic mechanisms. *Neuropsychopharmacology, 20*, 322-39.

[63] Paulus, M. P., Hozack, N. E., Zauscher, B. E., Frank, L., Brown, G. G., Braff, D. L. & Schuckit, M. A. (2002). Behavioral and functional neuroimaging evidence for prefrontal dysfunction in methamphetamine-dependent subjects. *Neuropsychopharmacology, 26*, 53-63.

[64] Bolla, K. I., Eldreth, D. A., London, E. D., Kiehl, K. A., Mouratidis, M., Contoreggi, C., Matochik, J. A., Kurian, V., Cadet, J. L., Kimes, A. S., Funderburk, F. R. & Ernst, M. (2003). Orbitofrontal cortex dysfunction in abstinent cocaine abusers performing a decision-making task. *Neuroimage, 19*, 1085-94.

[65] Fishbein, D., Hyde, C., Eldreth, D., London, E. D., Matochik, J., Ernst, M., Isenberg, N., Steckley, S., Schech, B. & Kimes, A. (2005). Cognitive performance and autonomic reactivity in abstinent drug abusers and nonusers. *Exp Clin Psychopharmacol, 13*, 25-40.

[66] Wesley, M. J., Hanlon, C. A. & Porrino, L. J. (2011). Poor decision-making by chronic marijuana users is associated with decreased functional responsiveness to negative consequences. *Psychiatry Res, 191*, 51-9.

[67] Le Berre, A. P., Rauchs, G., La Joie, R., Mezenge, F., Boudehent, C., Vabret, F., Segobin, S., Viader, F., Allain, P., Eustache, F., Pitel, A. L. & Beaunieux, H. (2012). Impaired decision-making and brain shrinkage in alcoholism. *Eur Psychiatry* (In Press).

[68] Li, X., Zhang, F., Zhou, Y., Zhang, M., Wang, X. & Shen, M. Decision-making deficits are still present in heroin abusers after short- to long-term abstinence. *Drug Alcohol Depend* (In Press).

[69] Cservenka, A. & Nagel, B. J. (2012). Risky decision-making: an FMRI study of youth at high risk for alcoholism. *Alcohol Clin Exp Res, 36*, 604-15

[70] Lovallo, W. R., Yechiam, E., Sorocco, K. H., Vincent, A. S. & Collins, F. L. (2006). Working memory and decision-making biases in young adults with a family history of alcoholism: studies from the Oklahoma family health patterns project. *Alcohol Clin Exp Res, 30*, 763-73.

[71] Goudriaan, A. E., Oosterlaan, J., de Beurs, E. & van den Brink, W. (2006). Psychophysiological determinants and concomitants of deficient decision making in pathological gamblers. *Drug Alcohol Depend*, *84*, 231-9.

[72] Lawrence, A. J., Luty, J., Bogdan, N. A., Sahakian, B. J. & Clark, L. (2009). Problem gamblers share deficits in impulsive decision-making with alcohol-dependent individuals. *Addiction*, *104*, 1006-15.

[73] Johnson, C. A., Xiao, L., Palmer, P., Sun, P., Wang, Q., Wei, Y., Jia, Y., Grenard, J. L., Stacy, A. W. & Bechara, A. (2008). Affective decision-making deficits, linked to a dysfunctional ventromedial prefrontal cortex, revealed in 10th grade Chinese adolescent binge drinkers. *Neuropsychologia*, *46*, 714-26.

[74] Goudriaan, A. E., Grekin, E. R. & Sher, K. J. (2011). Decision making and response inhibition as predictors of heavy alcohol use: a prospective study. *Alcohol Clin Exp Res*, *35*, 1050-7.

[75] Xiao, L., Bechara, A., Gong, Q., Huang, X., Li, X., Xue, G., Wong, S., Lu, Z. L., Palmer, P., Wei, Y., Jia, Y. & Johnson, C. A. (2012) Abnormal Affective Decision Making Revealed in Adolescent Binge Drinkers Using a Functional Magnetic Resonance Imaging Study. *Psychol Addict Behav*. In press.

[76] Ernst, M., Grant, S. J., London, E. D., Contoreggi, C. S., Kimes, A. S. & Spurgeon, L. (2003). Decision-making in adolescents with behavior disorders and adults with substance abuse. *Am J Psychiatry*, *160*, 33–40.

[77] van Honk, J., Hermans, E. J., Putman, P., Montagne, B., Schutter, D. J. (2002). Defective somatic-markers in subclinical psychopathy. *Neuroreport*, *13*, 1025–7.

[78] Franklin, T. R., Acton, P. D., Maldjian, J. A., Gray, J. D., Croft, J. R., Dackis, C. A., O'Brien, C. P. & Childress, A. R. (2002). Decreased gray matter concentration in the insular, orbitofrontal, cingulate, and temporal cortices of cocaine patients. *Biol. Psychiatry*. *51*, 134–42.

[79] Cowan, R. L., Lyoo, I. K., Sung, S. M., Ahn, K. H., Kim, M. J., Hwang, J., Haga, E., Vimal, R. L., Lukas, S. E., Renshaw, P. F. (2003). Reduced cortical gray matter density in human MDMA (Ecstasy) users: a voxel-based morphometry study. *Drug Alcohol Depend*, *72*, 225-35.

[80] Tanabe, J., Tregellas, J. R., Dalwani, M., Thompson, L., Owens, E., Crowley, T. & Banich, M. (2009). Medial orbitofrontal cortex gray matter is reduced in abstinent substance-dependent individuals. *Biol Psychiatry*, *65*, 160-4.

[81] Churchwell, J. C., Lopez-Larson, M. & Yurgelun-Todd, D. A. (2012). Altered frontal cortical volume and decision making in adolescent cannabis users. *Front Psychol*, *1*, 225.

[82] Moreno-López, L., Catena, A., Fernández-Serrano, M. J., Delgado-Rico, E., Stamatakis, E. A., Pérez-García, M. & Verdejo-García, A. (2012). Trait impulsivity and prefrontal gray matter reductions in cocaine dependent individuals. *Drug Alcohol Depend*, *125*, 208-14.

[83] Lim, K. O., Choi, S. J., Pomara, N., Wolkin, A., Rotrosen, J. P. (2002). Reduced frontal white matter integrity in cocaine dependence: a controlled diffusion tensor imaging study. *Biol. Psychiatry*, *51*, 890–5.

[84] Lyoo, I. K., Streeter, C. C., Ahn, K. H., Lee, H. K., Pollack, M. H., Silveri, M. M., Nassar, L., Levin, J. M., Sarid-Segal, O., Ciraulo, D. A., Renshaw, P. F. & Kaufman, M. J. (2004). White matter hyperintensities in subjects with cocaine and opiate dependence and healthy comparison subjects. *Psychiatry Res*, *131*, 135–45.

[85] Schlaepfer, T. E., Lancaster, E., Heidbreder, R., Strain, E. C., Kosel, M., Fisch, H. U. & Pearlson, G. D. (2006). Decreased frontal white-matter volume in chronic substance abuse. *Int J Neuropsychopharmacol*, *9*, 147-53.

[86] Chung, A., Lyoo, I. K., Kim, S. J., Hwang, J., Bae, S. C., Sung, Y. H., Sim, M. E., Song, I. C., Kim, J., Chang, K. H. & Renshaw, P. F. (2007). Decreased frontal white-matter integrity in abstinent methamphetamine abusers. *Int J Neuropsychopharmacol*, *10*, 765-75.

[87] Paulus, M. P., Hozack, N., Frank, L., Brown, G. G. & Schuckit, M. A. (2003). Decision making by methamphetamine-dependent subjects is associated with error-rate-independent decrease in prefrontal and parietal activation. *Biol Psychiatry*, *53*, 65-74.

[88] Tanabe, J., Thompson, L., Claus, E., Dalwani, M., Hutchison, K., Banich, M. T. (2007). Prefrontal cortex activity is reduced in gambling and nongambling substance users during decision-making. *Hum. Brain Mapp*, *28*, 1276–86.

[89] Grant, S., London, E., Newlin, D. B., Villemagne, V. L., Liu, X., Contoreggi, C., Phillips, R. I., Kimes, A. S. & Margolin, A. (1996). Activation of memory circuits during cue-elicited cocaine craving. *Proc. Natl. Acad. Sci. U.S.A.*, *93*, 2040–5.

[90] Sell, L. A., Morris, J. S., Bearn, J., Frackowiak, R. S. J., Friston, K. J., Dolan, R. J. (2000). Neural responses associated with cue evoked emotional states and heroin in opiate addicts. *Drug Alcohol Depend*, *60*, 207–16.

[91] Tapert, S. F., Brown, G. G., Baratta, M. V. & Brown, S. A. (2004). fMRI BOLD response to alcohol stimuli in alcohol dependent young women. *Addict Behav*, *29*, 33–50.

[92] Wrase, J., Grüsser, S. M., Klein, S., Diener, C., Hermann, D., Flor, H., Mann, K., Braus, D. F. & Heinz, A. (2002). Development of

alcoholassociated cues and cue-induced brain activation in alcoholics. *Eur Psychiatry*, *17*, 287–91

[93] Grusser, S. M., Wrase, J., Klein, S., Hermann, D., Smolka, M. N., Ruf, M., Weber-Fahr,W., Flor, H., Mann, K., Braus, D. F. & Heinz, A. (2004). Cue-induced activation of the striatum and medial prefrontal cortex is associated with subsequent relapse in abstinent alcoholics. *Psychopharmacology (Berl.)*, *175*, 296–302.

[94] Filbey, F. M., Schacht, J. P., Myers, U. S., Chavez, R. S., Hutchison, K. E. (2009). Marijuana craving in the brain. *Proc Natl Acad Sci USA*, *106*, 13016-21.

[95] Bechara, A. & Martin, E. M. (2004). Impaired decision making related to working memory deficits in individuals with substance addictions. *Neuropsychology*, *18*, 152-62.

[96] Kübler, A., Murphy, K. & Garavan, H. (2005). Cocaine dependence and attention switching within and between verbal and visuospatial working memory. *Eur J Neurosci*, *21*, 1984 –92.

[97] George, O., Mandyam, C. D., Wee, S. & Koob, G. F. (2008). Extended access to cocaine self-administration produces long-lasting prefrontal cortex dependent working memory impairments. *Neuropsychopharmacology*, *33*, 2474 –82.

[98] Verdejo, A., Aguilar de Arcos, F. & Pérez-García, M. (2004). Alteraciones de los procesos de toma de decisiones vinculados al cortex prefrontal ventromedial en pacientes drogodependientes. *Rev Neurol*, *38*, 601-606.

[99] DiClemente, C. C. (2007). Mechanisms, determinants and processes of change in the modification of drinking behavior. *Alcohol Clin Exp Res*, *31*(Suppl), 13s-20s.

In: Prefrontal Cortex
Editors: R. O. Collins and J. L. Adams
ISBN 978-1-62618-663-7

Chapter 3

PREFRONTAL CORTEX DYSFUNCTION AND NEUROCOGNITIVE DEFICITS IN SCHIZOPHRENIA: TARGETS OF OPPORTUNITY

Savita G. Bhakta* and Neal R. Swerdlow
Department of Psychiatry, UCSD School of Medicine, La Jolla, CA, US
VISN-22 MIRECC, VA HealthCare System, San Diego, CA, US

ABSTRACT

Several lines of evidence suggest that pathological alterations in specific neuronal circuits within the prefrontal cortex (PFC), including those inter-connecting the PFC and the mesial temporal lobe, may result in impaired neurocognitive functioning in schizophrenia (SZ) patients. These pathological alterations are thought to arise via disturbances in early neurodevelopmental and neural migratory processes, and ultimately degrade the efficiency of neural networks and thereby impair cognition. Recent reports have identified different neural substrates that are impacted by these aberrant neurodevelopmental processes, and these substrates are being explored as potential targets for pro-cognitive pharmacologic interventions in SZ. A number of cognitive, behavioral and pharmacological interventions modestly enhance neurocognitive

* Correspondence: Savita G. Bhakta, M.D., Department of Psychiatry, UCSD School of Medicine, 9500 Gilman Dr., La Jolla, CA 92093-0804, sgbhakta@ucsd.edu, 619-543-7109.

function to some degree in SZ patients. Here, we consider opportunities for optimizing PFC performance, to enable residual healthy circuitry to maximize benefits from these interventions, and thereby improve neurocognition in SZ.

Intrinsic and extrinsic processes may contribute to suboptimal PFC function in SZ, and may provide opportunities for interventions that optimize PFC performance. Such intrinsic factors include specific genes, circadian rhythm disturbances, and metabolic impairments; extrinsic factors include medications, nutrition and substance use. To the degree that these factors are correctable, they may prove to moderate the success of pharmacological and cognitive interventions aimed at optimizing real-life function in SZ.

Keywords: Prefrontal cortex, neurocognition, cognitive impairment, schizophrenia

1. INTRODUCTION

The importance of the prefrontal cortex (PFC) in neuropsychiatry stems from its critical role in governing and executing neurocognitive and emotional processes. The extensive interconnectivity between PFC and much of the brain, including other cortical, subcortical and brain stem sites allows it to contribute widely to the regulation of higher order functions (Wise SP et al., 1996; Fuster JM, 1989; Miller EK, 1999). Alterations in PFC connections arising from aberrant neurodevelopmental processes have been implicated in the pathophysiology of neurocognitive deficits in schizophrenia (SZ) (Barbas and Pandya, 1991; Cohen and Servan-Schreiber, 1992).

SZ is a debilitating mental illness affecting 1% of the general population and is characterized by positive and negative symptoms and neurocognitive deficits. Neurocognitive deficits are a core feature of this illness, and are known to predict functional outcome in SZ patients (Weinberger et al., 1986; cf. Barch, 2005; Keedy et al., 2006; Keefe et al., 2006a). However, medications currently available to treat SZ diminish positive symptoms, and to a lesser extent negative symptoms, but have little or no beneficial effect on neurocognitive symptoms. A growing interest in developing pro-cognitive treatment strategies has broadened our knowledge about the neurobiology and neurochemistry of PFC related neurocognitive deficits. In addition, sensitive instruments to measure these neurocognitive deficits and pro-cognitive treatment outcomes have been validated in humans as well as across species (Green et al., 2004a; Carter and Barch et al., 2007)

Applications of these tools and basic knowledge towards developing pro-cognitive drugs are in their initial stages. Results from clinical and translational research using pharmacological agents such as d-serine, d-amphetamine (AMPH) and modafinil have shown inconsistent cognitive enhancing effects (Barch and Carter, 2005; Kantrowitz et al 2010; Kane et al., 2010; Pietrzak et al., 2010a,b; Bobo et al., 2011; Scoriels et al., 2012; Dawson et al., 2012; Weiser et al., 2012; Chou et al., 2013; Müller et al., 2013). On the other hand, cognitive and behavioral treatment strategies such as the cognitive and social skills training and computer based Targeted Cognitive Training (TCT) have proven to be successful in reducing neurocognitive deficits and improving functional outcome (Twamley et al., 2008; McGurk et al., 2009; Medalia and Choi, 2009; Vinogradov, 2012a; b), albeit in some cases with modest effect sizes (Wykes et al., 2011).

Given the modest impact of these interventions, it becomes necessary to recognize the factors interfering with PFC functioning that are independent of the illness per se, and to optimize PFC functioning by targeting residual healthy neural circuitry to maximize clinical benefits. For example, attention/vigilance is a PFC based cognitive process, defined as the ability to allocate and sustain a focus of cognitive resources on specific stimuli or information, while ignoring distractors (Parsuraman, 1998). Impairment in attention may impact other cognitive processes such as learning, memory and cognitive flexibility, and importantly, may limit the utility of cognitive therapies for SZ. Thus, attentional impairment resulting from correctable factors such as circadian rhythm disturbances and anticholinergic or benzodiazepines medications should be addressed as a means to optimize clinical benefits from attention-dependent therapies.

This chapter reviews factors that interfere with PFC functioning in SZ patients, grouped into those that are "intrinsic" vs. "extrinsic;" strategies to identify and treat some of these correctable factors are illustrated as well. Recognition of these factors in the design of pro-cognitive research studies will help minimize potential experimental confounds, and more importantly, early identification and treatment of these factors may improve clinical outcome in SZ patients.

2. Neuropathology of the PFC and Neurocognitive Deficits in SZ

Because, PFC is the first neocortical brain region to arise in the neural tube and the last to complete maturation, it is highly susceptible to disruption (Ghika, 2008; Stiles and Jernigan, 2010). The U-shaped pattern of development of PFC gray matter - with growth in early childhood, pruning in adolescence and then slight growth and stabilization in adulthood - is linked with maturation of cortical circuits that underlie PFC functioning (Lenroot and Giedd, 2006). Maturing connections between PFC and other brain regions are positively correlated with development of age-appropriate cognitive abilities and behavior (Olesen et al., 2003; Nagy et al., 2004). For example, the development of connectivity between the PFC and parietal lobes is credited with the genesis of working memory capacity. Several other higher order cognitive processes such as flexible, decision-making (Lee et al., 2007), top-down regulation of attention (Knight et al., 1995; Buschman and Miller, 2007) and sensorimotor gating measured by prepulse inhibition (Bubser and Koch, 1994; Ellenbroek et al., 1996; Arime et al., 2012) all rely on PFC maturation and interconnectivity with other brain regions.

Alterations in PFC development or maturation of cortical connectivity are strongly implicated in the neuropathology of SZ. Animal models of SZ have shown that early exposure to stress, or neonatal ventral hippocampal lesions, impact peri-adolescent maturation of PFC neuronal circuits and are accompanied by the development of SZ-like cognitive deficits and behavior (Gruber et al., 2010; Markham et al., 2012; O'Donnell, 2012). Both neuro-pathological and structural neuroimaging studies in humans have revealed reduction in PFC volume in SZ patients (Pierri et al., 2001; Arnsten, 2011; Sapara et al., 2007; cf. Honea et al., 2005). In addition, functional neuroimaging studies have found either increased or decreased activation of PFC with respect to the difficulty level of the cognitive task in SZ patients (Dreher et al., 2012, Grillon et al., 2012). Patterns of aberrant connections, both within the PFC and between the PFC and other brain regions, can predict to some extent the severity of cognitive deficits in SZ patients (Cole et al., 2011).

Patients with SZ exhibit profound deficits in working memory, inhibitory control, social cognition, decision-making and set shifting, all of which are essential for everyday functioning, including the ability to maintain and build social relationships. However these deficits are highly variable among patients, making it difficult to design a "generic" pro-cognitive treatment regimen. Hence, identification of neurobiological "markers" for "sensitive" patient subgroups will facilitate the development of targeted effective pro-cognitive treatments.

3. Neural Substrates in the PFC: Potential Targets for Pro-Cognitive Pharmacologic Intervention

The neurochemical environment of PFC is rich with neurotransmitters, some of which may be targets for pharmacologic interventions to optimize PFC function. Specific examples are discussed below:

3.1. Dopamine (DA)

The functioning of PFC is highly sensitive to modulation by DA activity. DA is a major neuromodulator produced by neurons whose cell bodies are located in the midbrain, and which project to large areas of brain, including the dorsal and ventral striatum and the PFC (Swanson, 1982). Depletion or blockade of DA neurotransmission in the PFC is associated with impaired performance in numerous measures, including working memory and delayed response tasks (Brozoski et al., 1979; Sawaguchi et al., 1990 a,b). In SZ, a dysregulation of DA physiology has long been hypothesized. For example, dysregulation of DA signaling in SZ was proposed by Carter and Pycock (1980), with increased mesolimbic DA activity responsible for positive symptoms, and decreased mesocortical DA activity responsible for negative symptoms and cognitive deficits (cf. Deutch, 1992). Functional magnetic resonance imaging (fMRI) studies have shown positive associations between low levels of PFC DA and impaired performance on working memory tasks (Barch, 2003). The currently available antipsychotics are either potent DA antagonists or a mix of DA and serotonin receptor antagonists, that are effective in treating positive symptoms but are relatively ineffective in treating negative symptoms or cognitive deficits (Lieberman et al., 2005; Leucht et al., 2009).

DAergic transmission involves an inter-play among DA receptors, enzymes that metabolize DA in the synaptic cleft and DA transporters (DAT).

The DA receptors are grouped into families of DA1-like receptors (D1 and D5) and DA2-like receptors (D2, D3 and D4). The dynamics of DA within the PFC are dependent on the interactions among these components, which in turn may be regulated by endogenous (genetic) or exogenous (medication) processes.

Opportunities for Procognitive Interventions

DA agonists- Direct DA agonists bind to DA receptors, while indirect agonists enhance DAergic transmission via increasing DA release and/or blocking DA reuptake or catabolism. AMPH and methylphenidate are indirect DA agonists that are FDA approved for treatment of attention deficit hyperactivity disorder (ADHD). Several lines of evidence have shown enhanced cognitive performance with AMPH in SZ and SZ spectrum patients (Table 1). Individual studies examining the cognitive enhancing effects of AMPH in antipsychotic-medicated SZ patients have found AMPH to improve neurocognition without exacerbating psychotic symptoms (Goldberg et al., 1991; Barch and Carter, 2005; Pietrzak et al., 2010a,b). Likewise, both methylphenidate (Elliott et al., 1997; Mehta et al., 2004) and the direct D2-agonist, bromocriptine (Kimberg et al., 1997), have been reported to enhance PFC-based neurocognitive measures in healthy subjects (HS), but neither of these drug effects on neurocognition are well studied in SZ patients. In antipsychotic-medicated SZ, and SZ-spectrum patients, direct DA agonists such as pergolide and pramipexole have demonstrated variable effects on cognition (Sekine et al., 2005; McClure et al., 2010; Kelleher et al., 2012). While direct stimulation of D1 receptors in PFC may ultimately prove most effective in enhancing neurocognition in SZ, studies using the full direct D1 agonist, dihydrexidine, remain in progress (George et al. 2007).

Catechol-O-methyltransferase (COMT) is an enzyme that metabolizes DA and it is the primary mechanism of degrading DA in the PFC. Tolcapone is a centrally acting, reversible, selective COMT inhibitor approved for treatment of Parkinson's disease (Roche, 1998). Several research groups have reported, enhanced neurocognitive performance with tolcapone administration in healthy individuals who have relatively increased COMT enzyme activity and presumed low basal PFC DA tone based on the COMT Val/Val rs4680 genotype, (Apud et al., 2007; Giakoumaki et al., 2008). Tolcapone's effects on neurocognition, in SZ patients are not yet reported.

Table 1. Amphetamine effects in antipsychotic- medicated SZ and SZ spectrum patients

Study	Population	N	Dose (po)	*Δ performance*	Measure	* AE
Goldberg et al., 1991	SZ	21	0.25 mg/kg	+	Wisconsin Card Sorting Task (WCST), Trails-B	no
Barch & Carter, 2005	SZ	10	0.25 mg/kg	+	Spatial working memory (WM), language production	no
Pietrzak et al., 2010 a	SZ	32	10 mg	+	CogState: SP, A/V, R/PS*	no
Pietrzak et al., 2010 b	SZ	24	20 mg	+	R/PS	no
Siegel et al., 1996	SZ spectrum	9	30 mg	+	WCST	no
Study	population	N	Dose (po)	*Δ performance*	measure	* AE
Kirrane et al., 2000	SZ spectrum	12	30 mg	+	Visuospatial WM	no
Wonodi et al., 2006	SZ spectrum	11	30mg (twice)	+	Antisaccade latency	no

* AE: Adverse events; SP: speed of processing; A/V: attention/vigilance; R/PS: Reasoning/Problem Solving.

Clearly, the use of DA agonists such as AMPH to treat neurocognitive symptoms in SZ challenges the simplest interpretation of the "DA hypothesis of SZ" (van Rossum, 1966; Randrup and Munkvad, 1967). According to this simplest view, DA agonists such as AMPH should exacerbate psychosis, based on the accepted causal connection of DA hyperfunction and psychosis in SZ (Snyder, 1973); repeated dosing with DA agonists should precipitate psychotic symptoms in otherwise healthy individuals, based on the emergence of psychosis in stimulant abusers. A more discerning view of this dogma is that: 1) neurocognitive and other symptoms associated with functional impairment in SZ may actually reflect prefrontal DA hypofunction (cf. Kuepper et al., 2012), correctable with pro-DAergic drugs, and which is linked experimentally to genetic polymorphisms associated with high activity forms of COMT, the enzyme responsible for most PFC DA catabolism (Egan et al., 2001); 2) empirically, oral administration of AMPH to SZ– and SZ-spectrum patients is associated with modest neurocognitive improvement and not symptom exacerbation (Table 1). What Barch & Carter (2005) observed in their studies is echoed across the reports by other investigators: "individuals with SZ did not show an increase in symptoms, either positive or negative, with AMPH." 3) controlled, stable dose regimens of oral AMPH and other DA agonists are widely prescribed for ADHD and other conditions without a propensity for precipitating psychosis or abuse (Rapoport et al., 1980). Even in disorders viewed to reflect DA hyperfunction (e.g. Tourette Syndrome), AMPH and other DA agonists have therapeutic rather than adverse effects (Kurlan, 2003); 4) pro-DAergic drugs such as amantadine have long been used in AP-medicated SZ patients without evidence of psychotic exacerbation; and 5) a review of the use of AMPH in community-based AP-medicated SZ patients reveals it to be associated with reduced negative symptoms and no changes in positive symptoms (Nolte et al., 2004). Perhaps most importantly, a proposed use for DA agonists to selectively augment the therapeutic impact of cognitive interventions in SZ (discussed below) would limit the total exposure of SZ patients to these drugs, which could be administered under clinical supervision, within an integrated treatment model.

3.2. Glutamate

Glutamate is a widely distributed excitatory neurotransmitter. Convergent evidence suggests that glutamate dysfunction might play a primary role in SZ pathophysiology, based on the neurobehavioral and neurocognitive symptoms produced by non-competitive N-methyl D-aspartate (NMDA) antagonists such as phencyclidine (PCP) and ketamine (Javitt, 1987; Tamminga et al., 1995; Coyle, 1996; Abi-Saab et al., 1998; Olney et al., 1999; Jentsch and Roth, 1999; Newcomer et al., 1999). Glutamate receptors are classified into two broad families: 1) the ionotropic receptor family is comprised of NMDA, AMPA and kainate receptors, and 2) the metabotropic receptor (mGluR) family is G-protein coupled and mediates longer-term neuromodulatory effects of glutamate (Pin and Acher, 2002).

NMDA receptors are primarily sensitive to glutamate, however the allosteric modulatory sites for these receptors are sensitive to endogenous brain amino acids, glycine and d-serine. The glycine-binding site regulates channel open time and desensitization rate in the presence of agonist (glutamate), but does not, of itself, induce channel opening. AMPA receptors have an important role in long-term potentiation (LTP), a fundamental process necessary for learning, memory and synaptic plasticity (Miyamoto, 2006). However, both AMPA and kainate receptors work in synergy with NMDA receptors, and dysfunction in any one of these receptors impacts the functioning of other receptors. The mGLUR(s) regulate presynaptic glutamate release and postsynaptic sensitivity. Glycine transporters (GLYT) are present on neuronal membranes and reabsorb glycine, which is important for NMDA receptor functioning (Javitt, 2007).

Opportunities for Pro-Cognitive Interventions

NMDA receptor glycine-site agonists: While NMDA and AMPA receptors cannot be directly targeted with agonists for risk of inducing seizures, excitotoxicity and cortical hyperexcitability, the allosteric binding sites on PFC NMDA receptors are considered as potential targets for enhancing cognition. Studies conducted with glycine (30–60 g/day dose) (Heresco-Levy et al., 1999; Evins et al., 2000; Javitt et al., 2001; Heresco-Levy et al., 2004) and D-serine (2.1 g/day dose) (Tsai et al.,1998, 1999; Heresco-Levy et al., 2005; Weiser et al., 2012), which function as full agonists at the glycine binding site, have yielded inconsistent results in SZ patients. One study (Tsai et al., 2005) with D-alanine (7 g/day dose), a close structural analogue of D-serine, showed positive cognitive enhancing effects. Ongoing studies with D-cycloserine added to antipsychotics suggest limited benefits on select neurocognitive tasks, and perhaps an ability to enhance the impact of cognitive-behavioral therapy on delusional intensity (Goff et al. 2008b; Gottlieb et al. 2011).

AMPA receptor agonists: AMPAkines are positive allosteric modulators of the AMPA receptors. In both human (Ingvar et al., 1997) and animal (Hampson, 1998a, b) models they may facilitate learning and memory by desensitizing AMPA receptors. AMPAkine CX-516 significantly improved memory and attention when added to clozapine in a pilot study (Goff et al., 2001), but other studies failed to show any neurocognitive benefits (Marenco et al., 2002; Goff et al. 2008a).

Metabotropic glutamate receptor (mGluR) agonists: Agonists of mGluR(s) regulate presynaptic glutamate release. Several high-affinity agonists have been developed and tested in clinical and preclinical studies over recent years, including LY379268 and the related compound LY354740 (Schoepp and Marek, 2002). In preclinical animal studies, LY379268 was found to reverse PCP induced working memory impairment (Moghaddam and Adams, 1998; Lorrain et al., 2003). Likewise, LY354740 has been found to improve working memory deficits during ketamine infusion in otherwise healthy humans (Krystal et al., 2005).

Other Agents: Memantine, an NMDA partial antagonist approved for treatment of dementia, is being explored as a procognitive agent for SZ. Although NMDA hypofunction is implicated in producing SZ-like behavioral effects, the neurocognitive deficits in SZ have been proposed by some to be caused by glutamatergic hyperactivity in the PFC (Deutsch et al., 2001). In a double-blind randomized controlled trial (RCT), memantine (20 mg) failed to show any significant pro-cognitive effects in SZ patients (Lee et al., 2012), though other reports suggest pro-cognitive effects of memantine in SZ patients (de Lucena et al., 2011) and in patients with bipolar disorder (Teng and Demetrio, 2006; Iosifescu et al., 2012).

3.3. Acetylcholine (ACh)

Cholinergic system dysfunction in SZ has been proposed based on the behavioral and cognitive effects of anticholinergic drugs (Mego et al., 1988; Sarter et al., 2005). ACh is known to have a functional role in conscious awareness and components of information processing, including attention, working memory, encoding, memory consolidation and retrieval (Perry et al., 1999; Gold, 2003). The M1, M2 and M4 subtypes of muscarinic cholinergic receptors (mAChR) are widely distributed in the brain, with high concentrations in hippocampus and PFC, and are thought to play an important role in sensorimotor gating, learning, memory and synaptic plasticity (cf. Volipicelli and Levey, 2004). Likewise the nicotinic AChR subtypes, alpha 4 beta 2 ($\alpha_4\beta_2$) and alpha 7 (α_7) are thought to play an important role in regulating cognitive processes, and are reduced in SZ patients (Levin et al., 2006; Perl et al., 2006). Deficits in cholinergic receptors and neurotransmitter in the forebrain and its projections are implicated in the cognitive dysfuntion in SZ patients.

Opportunities for Procognitive Interventions

Acetylcholinesterase inhibitors (ChEI)s: These drugs such as donepezil, rivastigmine and galantamine- inhibit the enzyme ChE and thus increase the ACh concentration in the brain, and are already approved for the treatment of dementia (Rees and Brimijoin, 2003). However, data from RCTs and open-label trials with these drugs in SZ patients to enhance cognition remain inconclusive (Ribeiz et al., 2010; Lindenmayer and Khan, 2011; Singh et al., 2012).

M1 receptor allosteric agonists and positive allosteric modulators (PAM): VU0357017 is a highly potent, selective, and systemically active third-generation M1 allosteric agonist (Lebois et al., 2010). It activates the M1 mAChR at a novel allosteric site and blocks scopolamine-induced deficits in contextual fear conditioning (Lebois et al., 2010). Likewise, benzylquinolone carboxylic acid (BQCA), a systemically active and selective M1 PAM, reverses scopolamine-induced disruptions of the hippocampus-mediated memory task of contextual fear conditioning and increases wakefulness, and restores deficits in mPFC-dependent discrimination reversal learning in a transgenic mouse (Ma et al., 2009; Shirey et al., 2009). Taken together, studies with M1 allosteric agonists and PAMs report that selective activation of M1 produces efficacy in preclinical models of cognitive enhancement and suggest a potential role for M1 activation in the enhancement of PFC-dependent synaptic plasticity and learning.

nAChR agonists: The α_7nAChR has been widely studied as a potential target for cognitive enhancement in SZ (Martin et al., 2004). DMXB-A is an alpha7-selective agonist that was reported to enhance cognitive performance in SZ patients in a proof of principle study (Olincy et al., 2006), but failed to enhance performance on MATRICS Consensus Cognitive Battery (MCCB) in a phase II clinical trial (Freedman et al., 2008).

Clinical studies targeting the $\alpha_4\beta_2$ nAChR have shown some positive results. Nicotine is a full agonist at the $\alpha_4\beta_2$ nAChR (Ochoa et al., 1990; Flores et al., 1992) and is widely used by SZ patients (Hughes et al., 1986; cf. Leonard et al., 2001; Poirier et al., 2002). Several preclinical and clinical studies have shown nicotine to improve performance on cognitive tasks in smokers following smoking cessation, and in non-smokers (Bell et al., 2002; Sacco et al., 2005; Rusted et al., 2006; Atzori et al., 2008; Evans and Drobes, 2009). Studies with nicotine replacements in SZ patients have also shown beneficial effects on cognitive performance (AhnAllen et al., 2008; Barr et al., 2008). The $\alpha_4\beta_2$ nAChR agonist, varenicline, improved performance on verbal learning and decreased the number of cigarettes smoked per day by SZ patients but, did not improve performance on any other cognitive tasks (Smith et al., 2009; Patterson et al., 2009).

3.4. Other Neurotransmitters

In addition to DA, glutamate and ACh, several other neural substrates are known to modulate PFC functioning and cognitive processes, some of which may present opportunities for pro-cognitive interventions, as discussed below:

3.4.a Norepinephrine (NE): NE and its role in PFC functioning and cognition has been studied across species (cf. Arnsten, 2004). Alpha (2A) adrenergic receptors are present on both pre- and post-synaptic terminals. The post-synaptic alpha 2A receptors are considered potential targets for cognitive enhancement (Coull, 1994). Clonidine, an alpha 2A agonist, was reported to improve performance on Trails B test (Fields et al., 1988), and normalize sensorimotor gating (Oranje and Glenthoj, 2012) in SZ patients; guanfacine and guanabenz may have better side-effect profiles, and improved performance on working memory tasks, a continuous performance task and stroop interference tests in ADHD and healthy human volunteers (Jakala et al., 1999 a, b; Newcomer et al., 1999; Scahill, 2001; Taylor and Russo, 2001). Adding guanfacine to atypical antipsychotics was reported to have some significant, and some trend-level benefits, on select neurocognitive tasks in SZ patients (Friedman et al., 2001).

3.4.b Serotonin: Of the (approximately) 14 known serotonin receptors, the 5-HT(1A) and 5-HT(7) receptors are candidates for mediating at least some 5-HT effects on cognition (Gary and Roth, 2007). 5-HT(1A) receptor stimulation and 5-HT (7) receptor antagonism result in DA efflux in the PFC, which might contribute to their impact on cognition (Millan, 2000). A series of studies involving the 5-HT(1A) partial agonists tandospirone (Sumiyoshi et al., 2000; Sumiyoshi et al., 2001 a, b) and buspirone (Sumiyoshi et al., 2007; Keefe et al., 2006b) have reported a modest ability of these agents to improve some domains of cognition in SZ patients receiving typical or atypical antipsychotic drugs. Lurasidone is an antipsychotic with D2, 5HT2A and 5HT7 receptor blocking properties (Nolan and Roman, 2012) that exhibits a pro-cognitive-like profile in animal model studies (Horisawa et al., 2013).

3.4.c. Gamma amino butyric acid (GABA): In postmortem studies, Lewis et al. (2005) reported an upregulation of GABA (A) receptors containing the a(2) subunit, localized to the axon initial segment of PFC pyramidal cells. This upregulation may reflect the loss of GABAergic inputs to these receptors. In a proof of principle study, the GABA (A) a(2)/a(3) partial agonist, MK-0777, improved delayed memory performance and decreased reaction times on several PFC related cognitive tasks (Lewis et al., 2008), but failed to show any improvement when tested in a large RCT (Buchanan et al., 2011).

3.4.d. Oxytocin: Oxytocin is a neuropeptide secreted by magnocellular cells in the supraoptic nucleus and stored in neurosecretory vesicles in the posterior pituitary. Reduced levels of oxytocin are reported in SZ patients, and have been implicated in social cognitive deficits in this disorder (Rosenfeld et al., 2011). In preclinical studies involving animals and humans, synthetic oxytocin was reported to reverse the social cognitive deficits produced by phencyclidine (PCP) (Feifel and Reza, 1999; Lee et al., 2005; Kosfeld et al., 2005; Domes et al., 2007). RCTs in SZ patients report that oxytocin reduced paranoia and improved social cognition (Feifel et al., 2010; Pedersen et al., 2011; Feifel et al., 2012; Averbeck et al., 2012).

4. LABORATORY BASED MEASURES TO DETECT PRO-COGNITIVE EFFECTS

It is essential to use sensitive tools that can accurately detect efficacy signals early in the drug development process, to minimize the considerable costs of this process (Tufts Center for the Study of Drug Development, 2006). These tools can help prioritize compounds that demonstrate clear CNS effects in translational behavioral, neurophysiological or neuroimaging paradigms, thereby decreasing the risk for expensive late-stage failures. The Measurement and Treatment Research to Improve Cognition in SZ (MATRICS) (Green et al., 2004a) and the Cognitive Neuroscience Treatment Research to Improve Cognition in Schizophrenia (CNTRICS) (Carter and Barch, 2008) are National Institute of Mental Health (NIMH) sponsored programs that provide recommendations for cognitive assessment in preclinical and clinical SZ trials.

4.1. MATRICS

Table 2. MATRICS Consensus Cognitive Battery (Green et al., 2004a; Nuechterlein et al., 2008)

Cognitive Domain	Test
Speed of Processing	Brief Assessment of Cognition in SZ (BACS): Symbol Coding Category Fluency: Animal Naming Trail Making Test: Part A
Attention/Vigilance	Continuous Performance Test- Identical Pairs (CPT-IP)
Working memory (non verbal) (verbal)	Weschler Memory Scale ®- 3 rd Ed. (WMS® -III): Spatial Span Letter-Number Span
Verbal Learning	Hopkins Verbal Learning Test- Revised (HVLT-R)
Visual Learning	Brief Visuospatial Memory Test- Revised (BVMT-R)
Reasoning and problem solving	Neuropsychological Assessment Battery® (NAB®): Mazes
Social Cognition	Mayer-Salovey-Caruso Emotional Intelligence Test (MSCEIT): Managing Emotions

The MATRICS was designed to facilitate the development of novel cognitive treatments, and to equip the pharmaceutical industry as well as the Food and Drug Administration (FDA) to accept cognition as a pharmaceutical target (Green et al., 2004b). The MATRICS process identified 7 candidate cognitive domains and tests based on expert opinion and analysis of existing literature (Kern et al., 2004; Nuechterlein et al., 2004). Their consensus opinion was that working memory, attention/vigilance, verbal learning and memory, visual learning and memory, reasoning and problem solving, speed of processing, and social cognition comprised the primary domains of cognitive deficits in SZ (Green et al., 2004a). A selected number of tests were used in a multisite pilot study, results from which provided the basis for the final selection of 10 tests (Table 2.) that covered the 7 cognitive domains; these tests now constitute the MATRICS Consensus Cognitive Battery (MCCB) (Nuechterlein et al., 2008). The MCCB has been accepted by the FDA as a primary outcome measure for clinical trials targeting cognition in SZ. The excellent test–retest and inter-site reliability, and construct validity of the MCCB makes it a powerful tool to detect cognitive change in repeated testing applications and allows it to serve as a cognitive reference point for nonintervention studies of SZ and related disorders. In addition, the normative data for the entire MCCB, stratified by gender, three age groups and three levels of education, makes it broadly representative of the US population (Kern et al., 2008).

4.2. CNTRICS

Developing sensitive and sensible cognitive tests for clinical trials in schizophrenia is an iterative process. During the last phase of MATRICS, the CNTRICS program was initiated to draw attention to tasks that are informed by cognitive neuroscience (CN). The aim was to develop specialized tasks that probe the function of specific cognitive processes and have translational potential across species (Carter and Barch, 2007). The approach of including of CN-informed tasks in cognitive trials in schizophrenia has two benefits. First, it will be sensitive to detect drug effects that only affect a specific cognitive process; second, it will allow rapid vertical translation from animal to human research and vice versa. Moreover, the neural targets of such tasks can be cross-validated through experiments in animals and functional neuroimaging in humans (Carter et al., 2008).

5. Cognitive Training

Although SZ was once considered a neurodegenerative disease, it is now believed that with intervention, healthy neural circuitry can be modified in an adaptive manner to restore function to some extent (Cramer et al., 2011). Dramatic examples of neuroplasticity are seen in the process of stroke rehabilitation, where regained function reflects adaptive changes in neural circuitry. An awareness of the potential for such neuroplasticity has led to the development of cognitive training strategies that aim to improve cognitive functioning and functional outcome in SZ patients (Wykes and van der Gaag, 2001). How these strategies change the neural network, and the extent to which these changes reflect processes from gene expression up to the organization of circuits and systems, are questions of ongoing investigation (de Lange et al., 2008; Fox, 2009; Keller and Just, 2009; Korosi and Baram, 2009; Porto et al., 2009; Saxena et al., 2009).

Cognitive training, also known as "remediation" or "rehabilitation," can be broadly classified into those using restorative vs. compensatory strategies. Restorative strategies are drills and practice exercises that are based on evidence for lifelong neuroplasticity (Eack et al., 2010). They may be delivered in various ways: as computerized exercises, or therapist guided paper/pencil exercises, or combined computer exercises with verbal discussion to link training exercises to everyday life. The compensatory strategy, by contrast, aims to enhance adaptive behavior and therefore enhance functioning by developing strategies to circumvent neurocognitive impairment (Twamley, 2010). These involve functional adaptation skills training, such as training in social skills and communication domains, transportation domains, etc.

Cognitive training packages can be general, covering all cognitive domains, or be specific to one cognitive domain, depending on the cognitive deficits observed in the patient. Cognitive training programs are typically administered for 2-3 hours per week for at least 3 months, and across a variety of formats have been shown to be safe and modestly effective for SZ, with effect sizes of about 0.4 (Wykes et al., 2011).

5.1. Computer-Assisted Cognitive Remediation (CACR)

There are several commercial cognitive training software packages available, and many have been tested in RCTs in SZ patients. Typically, these programs provide exercises that are multisensory, with unlimited repetitions;

programs automatically adjust in difficulty level as the patient progresses (Field et al., 1997; Medalia et al., 2001; Sartory et al., 2005). Most of the commercially available programs target the cognitive domains listed in the MCCB (Bracy, 1995; Marker, 2001). A meta-analysis of 16 RCTs evaluating the efficacy of CACR in improving cognition overall and in specific domains, showed that they enhance both general cognition (effect size=0.38) and specific cognitive domains, but with small effect sizes (Grynszpan et al., 2011). Most of the CACR programs have a top-down approach of targeting cognitive domains, however brain fitness program (e.g. BFP developed by PositScience, Inc.) is a computerized training program with drills and practice exercises using a bottom-up approach that engages early perceptual processes to sharpen the accuracy and fidelity of auditory information processing in SZ (Vinogradov, 2012a; b). Plastic changes in neural substrates that subserve early perceptual processing feed forward to enhance higher-order cognition including attention, working memory, and the encoding and retrieval of verbal information. With increasing demands on early perceptual processes, auditory information processing improves, generalizing to enhanced "downstream" performance in higher-order cognitive functions. After 50 hours of Targeted Cognitive Training (TCT), SZ patients show large effect size (d=0.86-0.89) gains in auditory-dependent cognitive domains (verbal learning and memory), global cognition and quality of life that persist for at least 6 months post-TCT (Fisher et al., 2010; Subramaniam et al., 2012). Although TCT is efficacious at the group level, there is wide variability in individual responses, and some patients show little or no benefit (Fisher et al., 2009; Murthy et al., 2012); furthermore, 50 hours of training may not be feasible for many patients or clinics. Conceivably, pharmacologically-enhanced attention and vigilance might augment and accelerate procedural learning, and its effects on higher cognitive processes; this might happen via "top-down" drug effects – helping patients sustain or direct attention towards TCT stimuli - rather than via effects on early sensory processing per se. There is a critical need to identify predictive markers of TCT sensitivity, and to determine whether pharmacologic interventions can augment and accelerate TCT benefits. Importantly, training effects on tone discrimination and higher order processes can be detected after a single session (Lovio et al., 2012), making it possible to assess acute drug effects on TCT performance in a placebo-controlled single dose cross-over design.

5.2. Therapist Guided Paper/Pencil Task

Cognitive remediation therapy (CRT) involves therapist guidance, and targets tasks of memory, complex planning, and problem solving using simple paper/pencil tests and small task equipment. The therapist also provides information-processing strategies and discusses the regulation, organization and monitoring of behavior for each task to minimize error. Although Ueland and Rund (2004) did not find any change in functioning or cognition in adolescents with early onset psychosis, a RCT demonstrated significant improvement on Wisconsin Card Sorting Task, lasting for at least three months in SZ patients who received therapist guided paper/pencil cognitive training (Wykes et al. 2007).

5.3. Combined Computer Exercises and Therapist Guidance

This strategy involves computer exercises targeting several cognitive domains, along with guidance from therapists. The therapist provides examples of verbal mediation, spaced repetition and rehearsal. Bowie et al. (2012) showed that SZ patients who underwent this combined strategy had enhanced cognition compared to the SZ patients who only received functional adaptation skills training. However, this strategy did not produce significant improvements in real-world behavior and social competence.

5.4. Compensatory Cognitive Training (CCT)

There are many cognitive training programs that use compensatory strategies such as the cognitive adaptation training (CAT) (Velligan et al., 2009), cognitive and behavioral social skills training (CBSST) (Granholm et al., 2007) and functional adaptation skills training (Patterson et al., 2006). The domains and strategies included in CCT are mentioned in Table 3 (Twamley et al, 2012). The efficiency of these strategies in SZ patients is variable (Pilling et al., 2002). However, a meta-analysis of 6 studies using some form of CCT showed effect sizes (d) ranging from 0.2 to 1.2, with greatest improvement in neuropsychological measures, followed by psychosocial functioning, and lastly symptom reduction (Medalia and Choi, 2009).

Table 3. Compensatory Cognitive Training (Twamley et al., 2012)

Domains	Strategies
Prospective memory	Calendar use; to-do lists; prioritizing tasks
Attention/vigilance	Eye contact, paraphrasing, asking questions during conversations
Learning and memory	Taking notes; association; chunking; categorization; visual imagery
Executive functioning	6-step problem solving method; self-talk and self-monitoring while problem solving; set shifting; set maintenance

5.5. Combination of the Above Strategies

Because most of the above-mentioned strategies have strengths and weaknesses, combinations of strategies that have most benefits in specific domains are being developed and tested. Some of these programs are the neurocognitive enhancement training (NET) (Bell et al., 2008), cognitive enhancement training (CET) (Eack et al., 2007), and problem solving and cognitive flexibility program (REPYFLEC) (Farreny et al., 2012). A systematic review (Kluwe-Schiavon et al., 2013) of 30 RCTs including individual and combination cognitive training strategies found the most improvement in executive functions and functional improvement for studies using a combination of restorative and compensatory strategies. A meta-analysis of 40 randomized, controlled trials of 2,104 patients (Wykes et al., 2011) showed a medium effect size (0.5) for cognitive performance as measured by standardized cognitive tasks, and a medium effect size (0.42) for psychosocial functioning as measured by the ability to obtain and work competitive jobs, quality of and satisfaction with interpersonal relationships, and ability to solve interpersonal problems. Effect sizes for cognition and functioning were maintained at follow-up. Notably, effects on more generalized psychosocial functioning were stronger in studies that provided adjunctive psychosocial rehabilitation, and when compensatory strategy training was provided in the context of psychosocial rehabilitation (Medalia and Saperstein, 2013). Obviously, the use of combination therapies complicates the process of understanding, at a mechanistic level, which specific therapeutic elements are most beneficial to individual patients. Thus, while these "packaged" interventions may have superior efficacy, they present some limitations and complexities as research tools.

6. Reasons for Sub-Optimal PFC Activity and Modest Treatment Response

Currently available cognitive enhancing strategies - both pharmacological and non-pharmacological - produce only small to modest effect size improvements in function and cognition in SZ. Because of this, strategies are being developed for pharmacologic augmentation of cognitive therapies (PACT) (Swerdlow, 2011; 2012). Specifically, PACT strategies pair drug that target particular cognitive domains (e.g. attention/vigilance) with cognitive therapies that access/put demands on those domains. A "proof of concept" for this approach is being developed and applied through the use of drugs that selectively enhance the therapeutic benefits of cognitive and behavioral interventions for anxiety disorders (Ressler et al., 2004). PACT development has been discussed in detail in recent reports (Swerdlow, 2011; Chou et al., 2012).

In addition to developing novel therapeutic strategies for enhancing PFC function, and hence cognition, in SZ, it is imperative to consider what factors might be contributing to suboptimal PFC function in SZ patients, and which thereby may limit the effectiveness of any pro-cognitive intervention. These factors can be characterized as "intrinsic" vs. "extrinsic," based on whether they are present with-in the patient or are introduced from outside, respectively. Some intrinsic factors include genetics, sleep-related issues, metabolic impairment, age, and reproductive and other hormones. Examples of extrinsic factors are medications, illicit substance use, nutritional deficiency and lifestyle habits. Most of these factors interact, and importantly, are either modifiable or correctable.

6.1. Intrinsic Factors

6.1.a. Genes: Several functional polymorphisms and haplotypes have been identified that modify PFC function by altering the DA or glutamate activity. Understanding the role of genetic variation and its effects on the PFC is essential, as it can inform development of pro-cognitive interventions, and influence the responses to these interventions.

Genes influencing DA activity: The most widely studied gene in this category is the COMT gene present on the long arm of chromosome 22. A common functional single nucleotide polymorphism (SNP) rs4680 occurs at codon 108/158, wherein valine (Val) is substituted for methionine (Met) resulting in a four-fold variation in the COMT enzyme activity: compared to Met homozygotes, Val homozygotes have 4 times higher COMT enzyme activity (Lotta et al., 1995), which is the primary mechanism of DA degradation in the PFC. Both SZ patients and healthy subjects (HS) with Val/Val genotype perform poorly on cognitive tasks when compared to the Met/Met patients or HS respectively (Bruder et al., 2005; Wang et al., 2010). Similarly, effects of variations in the dopamine receptor (DR) D2 gene SNP rs1076560 and the RAC-alpha serine/threonine-protein kinase (AKT1) gene SNP rs1130233 have been studied; individually, and in conjunction, these variations influence the DA signaling pathway and working memory functioning (Tan et al., 2009; 2012).

Genes influencing glutamate activity: Genetic variations in the metabotropic receptors, especially group III (GRM3), group VII (GRM7) and group VIII (GRM8), have been associated with SZ and neurocognitive impairments in this disorder (Harrison et al., 2008; Need et al., 2009). The gene encoding for dystrobrevin binding protein1 (DTNBP1) or dysbindin1 on chromosome 6p is reported to be a SZ risk gene (Williams et al., 2005). Reduced expression of DTNBP1 in PFC is associated with cognitive deficits, and may influence the severity of intellectual decline in SZ (Hallmayer et al., 2005; Burdick et al., 2006; 2007). Other genes in the glutamate system that influence PFC functioning are neuregulin (NRG1) SNP rs35753505 (Mechelli et al., 2008; Kircher et al., 2009; Krug et al., 2010), DISC1 (Raznahan et al., 2011) and D-amino acid oxidase (DAAO) (Goldberg et al., 2006).

6.1.b. Sleep-related issues: It is well known that insufficient sleep leads to day-time fatigue and impairment in cognitive functioning (Killgore, 2010). SZ patients often have sleep disturbances that could be part of the illness itself or independent of the illness. Insomnia in SZ is often associated with an exacerbation of psychotic symptoms. Sleep studies in SZ patients reveal non-rapid eye movement (NREM) sleep disturbances, particularly related to stage 3 and sleep spindles, and circadian rhythm disturbances with reduced levels of melatonin (Keshavan et al., 2011; Wulff and Joyce, 2011). Disturbances in sleep spindles were associated with impairment in cognitive performance, particularly in PFC-related tasks. A small study with 14 SZ patients showed that restoration of sleep with melatonin was associated with improved cognitive performance (Bromundt et al., 2011).

Another sleep related issue in SZ is obstructive sleep apnea syndrome (OSAS) (Winkelman, 2001). In a Japanese study of over 100 SZ patients, 19% were diagnosed with OSAS (Takahashi et al., 1998). Antipsychotic-induced weight gain (an extrinsic factor discussed below) increases the risk for OSAS (Winkelman, 2001; Wirshing et al., 2002). OSAS is further associated with apnea and resulting hypoxia, multiple night-time awakenings and day-time fatigue and sleepiness. SZ patients with comorbid OSAS have more impaired attention/vigilance, working memory and executive functions, compared to SZ patients without OSAS (Jaffe et al., 2006). Treatment of OSAS with continuous positive airway pressure (CPAP) for 2-months in a placebo-controlled trial improved performance on n-back tasks and partially normalized alterations in the task positive and default mode network activations, suggesting that such intervention early in the disease might prevent or slow the occurrence of irreversible damage (Prilipko et al., 2011; 2012). Modafinil is a FDA approved drug for treatment of OSAS, that promotes wakefulness and in one open-label pilot study, significantly improved scores on cognitive tasks and global functioning, and reduced fatigue in SZ patients (Rosenthal and Bryant, 2004).

6.1.c. Metabolic Impairment: Important metabolic disorders - diabetes mellitus (DM) and metabolic syndrome (MetS) - along with hypertension (HTN) have been independently linked to cognitive impairments in SZ (Dickinson et al. 2008; Friedman et al., 2010; Lindenmayer et al., 2012), presumably due – at least in part – to their negative impact on PFC function. MetS, also known as "Syndrome X," is a cluster of symptoms characterized by abdominal obesity, impaired glucose metabolism, elevated blood pressure and dysregulation of plasma lipids (Sacks, 2004). Although the etiology of MetS is not clearly elucidated, several contributing factors are identified, including antipsychotic medications, visceral obesity, insulin resistance, hormonal imbalances, stress and chronic inflammation. MetS can increase the risk for cardiovascular disease and non-insulin dependent DM (NIDDM).

In a large multi-site Clinical Antipsychotic Trials of Intervention Effectiveness (CATIE), 43% of SZ patients had MetS, with higher percentages in women. In 63% of those patients, MetS went untreated (McEvoy, 2005). Although CATIE did not find any significant association between MetS and cognitive deficits, a recent study by Lindemayer et al. (2012) reported that SZ patients without MetS performed significantly better than those with MetS on tasks of processing speed, working memory, attention/vigilance and problem solving/reasoning. Takayanagi et al. (2012) and Dickinson et al. (2008) reported a similar association in SZ patients with co-morbid DM: patients with co-morbid DM performed poorer than SZ only or non-SZ patients with DM on tasks of processing speed, attention/working memory, executive functioning and visuo-spatial memory Furthermore, SZ patients with untreated DM showed poorer overall cognitive performance and a significantly lower score in the domain of vigilance compared with SZ patients without DM.These impairments were further associated with the duration and age of onset of DM. Similarly, Freidman et al. (2010) reported that SZ patients with HTN performed more poorly on verbal memory task, compared to SZ patients without HTN.

6.1.d. Age: This unmodifiable factor is an important variable in studies of cognition and PFC function. A common understanding is that younger adults outperform older adults in overall cognitive scores. A similar association of age and cognitive performance is seen in SZ patients. However, the association of age and response to cognitive training has been inconsistent. Kontis et al (2013) found that individuals above 40 years of age showed poor benefits from cognitive training, when compared to adults below age 40, which was not associated with factors of cognitive reserve. In contrast, others have shown that older SZ patients had significant improvements in cognitive performance after cognitive remediation, perhaps reflecting the fact that these older subjects had more range for improvement (McGurk et al., 2007; Twamley et al., 2011).

6.1.e. Reproductive hormones: Estrogen, along with brain derived neurotropic factor (BDNF), are essential for synaptic plasticity and dendritic spine formation (Luine and Frankfurt, 2012), and might thus be an intrinsic factor of importance to the PFC. In women, levels of estrogen vary throughout the lifespan (Dohanich, 2002; Luine, 2008). Estrogen levels have been associated with sensorimotor gating and cognition: low levels of estrogen accompany reduced sensorimotor gating and poor performance on cognitive tasks (Swerdlow et al., 1997; Van den Buuse and Eikelis, 2001; Vaillancourt et al., 2002; Driscoll et al., 2012). In preclinical animal and human studies, estrogen replacement improved cognitive performance in ovariectomized female rats or women who had undergone menopause or ovariectomy (Gasbarri et al., 2012; Acosta et al., 2013). Female SZ patients have a high propensity for amenorrhea and menstrual cycle irregularities as a result of antipsychotic medications, or due to the illness (Seeman, 2011). Conceivably, these hormonal irregularities might contribute to "suboptimal" PFC functions that limit treatment responses. Estradiol is reported to increase BDNF levels in PFC and hippocampus, and is being investigated as a potential cognitive enhancer (Luine and Frankfurt, 2012).

6.1.f. Other hormones: Thyroid hormone is widely distributed in the brain and is known to have an important role in brain development. The pituitary-thyroid axis alters DA receptor sensitivity and concentration (Santos et al.,

2012). Low levels of triiodothyronine (T3) in the brain are associated with poor myelination and impaired cognitive performance (Ichioka et al., 2012). Both typical and atypical antipsychotic medications impact thyroid hormone levels either by a central or peripheral mechanisms. Adverse central effects on thyroid function can reflect deiodination and immunogenic changes, or secondary consequences of hyperprolactinemia. Peripherally, piperazine and piperidine compounds such as aripiprazole and quetiapine, are known to interfere with thyroid hormone metabolism in the liver, thus resulting in subclinical hypothyroidism (Bou Khalil and Richa, 2011). Routine assessment of thyroid function parameters can help identify and treat subclinical hypothyroidism. Another common endocrine symptom in SZ is polydipsia resulting from DM, diabetes insipidus (DI) or syndrome of inappropriate antidiuretic hormone (SIADH) secretion. Neuroleptics used in the treatment of SZ can potentially cause SIADH, DM or DI. Polydipsia can cause hyponatremia, which impairs PFC functioning. Torres et al (2009) evaluated neuropsychological functioning in 3 groups of SZ patients - polydipsic hyponatremic, polydipsic normonatremic, and nonpolydipsic normonatremic - and found that polydipsic hyponatremic patients performed poorer than others on overall cognitive tasks. Treating the cause of polydipsia and restricting water intake can normalize sodium levels, and presumably help optimize PFC function.

6.2. Extrinsic Factors

6.2.a. Medications: Antipsychotic medications reduce positive symptoms in SZ, but have several untoward side-effects that might impair quality of life, and that directly or indirectly might impair cognition and PFC function (Fujimaki et al., 2012; Awad and Voruganti, 2004). Antipsychotic medications can induce weight gain, and cause obesity, MetS, DM, OSAS and other medical disorders mentioned earlier that can impair PFC functioning (Newcomer, 2005; Heal et al., 2012). Anticholinergic medications such as benztropine, diphenhydramine and trihexyphenidyl used for treating neuroleptic-induced extra-pyramidal side-effects (EPS) can produce significant impairment in neurocognitive functioning (Xiang et al., 2007; Desmarais et al., 2012). Reducing the dose of antipsychotics to reduce EPS, thereby limiting the need for anticholinergics, help optimize cognitive function in SZ patients.

Normal brain DA neurotransmission is essential for reward mechanisms critical to learning and other higher order cognitive processes. DA blockade has been shown to impair both motivation and acquisition of learned responses. Thus, even independent of their effects on peripheral and central metabolic processes, antipsychotics can impair important cognitive functions via the blockade of basal forebrain DA neurotransmission. Clearly, such deleterious effects on motivation and learning can have negative consequence on measures of neurocognitive performance, and on the potential benefits of cognitive interventions in SZ. Balanced against these counter-therapeutic effects of antipsychotics is the clear evidence that active psychosis is a strong negative predictor of therapeutic response to cognitive therapies (Sitzer et al., 2008). Ultimately, clinical decisions regarding antipsychotic choice and dose must weigh these interacting factors and their impact on motivation, learning, neurocognition and the therapeutic benefits of cognitive therapy.

6.2.b. Nutrition: Poor nutrition and obesity are associated with impaired cognitive function and cardiovascular morbidity and mortality (Waldstein and Katzel, 2006). These associations with cognitive impairment are likely bidirectional: individuals with impaired cognition are prone to have more limited and unhealthy dietary and exercise habits, and poor nutrition and sedentary lifestyles may impair PFC function by creating suboptimal metabolic and vascular support.

Contributors to obesity in SZ patients include both poor dietary habits and sedentary lifestyles. Several epidemiological studies of dietary habits in SZ patients living in care settings (Gupta and Craig, 2009) or community dwellings (McCreadie, 2003; Henderson et al., 2006; Simonelli-Munoz et al., 2012) have reported that patients consume high levels of saturated fats via "fast foods" and low levels of fruits, vegetables, fish and polyunsaturated fatty acids (PUFA). A combination of these dietary habits, along with over-eating secondary to dysregulated satiety and perhaps reward circuitry leads to high rates of obesity and nutritional deficiency in this population (Wirshing, 2004; Elman et al., 2006). Dietary intake of saturated fats increases risk for cardiovascular disease and DM by increasing atherogenic lipids and glucose resistance. Lower levels of PUFA in particular, docosahexaenoic acid (DHA) and archadonic acid (AA) in SZ patients, are associated with poor cognitive performance (van der Kemp et al., 2012). To date, results from RCTs using omega 3 fatty acids, DHA and eicosapentaenoic acid (EPA) to improve cognitive performance in SZ patients have been inconsistent (cf. Kidd, 2007).

Antipsychotic medications can trigger and exacerbate weight gain and obesity via changes in the patterns of food intake by increasing appetite

(Bromel et al., 1998; Kinon et al., 2005) and the subsequent consumption of a "fast food" diet (Gothelf et al., 2002; Kane et al., 2004); this pattern converges with a sedentary lifestyle, which is promoted by antipsychotic-induced sedative and extrapyramidal side-effects, and by amotivation, which can be both a primary consequence of SZ and an iatrogenic consequence of medications. Social isolation and impaired social cognition caused by SZ further exacerbate this process, by limiting a patient's exposure to socially-promoted dietary variety, restricting the opportunities for healthy physical activity, and obviating the social motivational contribution to weight control and health maintenance.

Obviously, the interplay between dietary and exercise habits, antipsychotics and the endogenous consequences of SZ is a complex one, requiring a multi-tier interventional strategy. Modification of dietary habits with counseling alone did not appear to change waist circumference or reduce cardiovascular morbidity in SZ patients (McCreadie et al., 2005). However, a health promotion program characterized by a combination of an exercise regimen and dietary modification, reportedly improved physical activity and mental health functioning, and reduced waist circumference and negative symptoms in SZ patients after 9 months of participation in the study (Van Citters et al., 2010).

6.2.c. Substance use: There is a strong association between SZ and smoking (De Leon and Diaz, 2005); about 77 % of SZ patients smoke tobacco compared to 15% of general population (Poirier et al., 2002; Hughes et al., 2006). Smoking is associated with cardiovascular and cerebrovascular disease, impaired cardiac output and cerebral perfusion, and reduced treatment effectiveness; and these many factors converge to negatively impact PFC function and cognition in SZ patients (McCloughen, 2003; Goff et al., 2005).

Cannabis is the most commonly used illicit drug by SZ patients (Green et al., 2005). Epidemiological studies have suggested a strong association between cannabis use and increased risk for SZ (Arseneault et al., 2002; van Os et al., 2002; Zammit et al., 2002). Studies with intravenous delta-9 tetrahydrocannabinol (THC) (Morrison et al., 2009; D'Souza et al. 2004; D'Souza et al., 2005), or ad lib smoking of marijuana cigarette (Hunault et al., 2009) in healthy subjects and stable SZ patients have reported both psychotic exacerbation and worsening of cognitive performance. The exact neural mechanism for the THC- induced neurocognitive deficits is still a subject of research, although cannabinoid 1 receptor abnormalities in the PFC have been identified in SZ patients (Eggan et al., 2008). Despite these findings in provocation studies, a systematic review by Segev and Lev Ran (2012) of 19 studies found no consistent differences in cognitive symptoms among cannabis-using vs. non-using SZ patients across a vast range of domains (memory, attention and processing speed, executive functions, visuospatial, psychomotor and language): 11 studies reported superior cognitive functions among cannabis-users, 5 found minimal or no differences between groups, and 3 found superior cognitive functions among cannabis-non-users. These results might be explained by methodological differences between the studies in subject selection, cognitive measures, measures of cannabis use, additional drugs used, and clinical aspects of SZ.

Other drugs abused by SZ patients that impair PFC functioning are alcohol (Abernathy et al., 2010) and ecstasy (McCann et al., 2008). Co-occurring substance use disorder is common among patients with SZ, and its presence is associated with poor medication compliance, physical comorbidities and poor health, poor self-care, which ultimately contributes to impaired PFC functioning. Therefore, screening and assessment for substance use, and integrated treatment plans for dual diagnosis that can address both the substance use and the mental illness are recommended in order to provide accurate treatment, and optimize PFC function.

7. Examples of Optimizing PFC Function

Given the identified intrinsic and extrinsic contributors to PFC function, it is worth considering how these factors, might be manipulated in an attempt to optimize this function, and hence maximize the ability of the PFC to sub-serve normal cognition in SZ patients. Two examples are given here:

7.1. Example of Modifying Intrinsic Factors – Pharmacogenetics

As noted above, the common functional SNP rs4680 of the COMT gene moderates PFC function and treatment response. SZ patients homozygous for Val allele have high PFC COMT activity and presumably lower levels of available PFC DA; they also have worse cognitive performance and exhibit more negative symptoms compared to Met/Met patients (Wang et al., 2010). This genetic polymorphism creates an opportunity for a pharmacogenetic approach to SZ, in which a treatment choice is dictated by the patients' SNP identity. Thus, a drug that increases PFC DA availability – via promoting DA release or blocking catabolism - should have particular value in Val/Val patients. In studies with HS, the DA releaser AMPH enhanced working memory performance in Val/Val individuals, and impaired working memory performance in the Met/Met individuals (Mattay et al., 2003), though conflicting findings have been reported (Hamidovic et al., 2010). Similar effects were reported using the COMT inhibitor, tolcapone, in measures of working memory and sensorimotor gating (Apud et al., 2007; Giakoumaki et al., 2008). It is thus worth considering whether drugs that enhance PFC DAergic tone, either via increased release or reduced catabolism, might enhance neurocognitive function among antipsychotic-treated Val/Val SZ patients.

In this simplest model, where neurocognitive deficits in Val/Val SZ patients are opposed by a drug that enhances PFC DA tone, potential deleterious effects of drug-induced subcortical DA release will be blunted via D2 blockade by antipsychotic medications, which will cause a relatively weaker blockade of D1-predominant PFC DA receptors (Creese et al., 1976; Hall et al., 1994). This remains a speculative and not-systematically tested hypothesis, and some findings (Mattay et al. 2003; Giakoumaki et al. 2008) suggest that this strategy should be avoided in Met/Met patients. Conceivably, COMT inhibition with tolcapone in Val/Val *SZ* patients, used in combination with a low dose of a DA releaser, might serve to focus increased DA tone within the PFC (where COMT is most active (Egan et al., 2001)), producing maximal pro-cognitive effects while minimizing dose requirements.

7.2. Example of Modifying Extrinsic Factors

Medical contributors to PFC function in SZ can be addressed by modifying some of the extrinsic factors via primary prevention and secondary interventions. Prevention of obesity and related medical disorders is one example of such an approach. Lifestyle modifications such as initiation of healthy dietary habits, exercise regimens and scheduled activity during the day have been reported to benefit cognition and function in SZ patients (Hill and Bessesen, 2003; Wilson and Grundy, 2003 a,b). In a meta-analysis of behavioral and pharmacologic treatments for atypical antipsychotic-induced weight gain, nutritional counseling combined with exercise, was found to be most effective regimen (Das et al., 2012). The use of antipsychotics with a lower propensity for inducing MetS such as ziprasidone, lurasidone (Risbood et al., 2012), molindone or aripiprazole (Wang et al., 2013) may be of particular value for SZ patients who are overweight or have a genetic predisposition to obesity (Zimmerman et al., 2003). Baseline evaluation of blood pressure, waist circumference, BMI, blood glucose levels and lipids upon antipsychotic initiation, followed by regular monitoring of these indices as per American Psychiatric Association and American Diabetic Association (APA/ADA) guidelines (ADA and APA, 2004) is an efficient strategy for early detection and prevention of MetS and other accompanying medical disorders. The second tier management of medical co-morbidities involves the use of insulin or anti-diabetic medications to control blood glucose, anti-hypertensive agents to regulate blood pressure, and statins or cholesterol lowering drugs to lower low-density lipoproteins and triglycerides and increase high-density lipoproteins. Obviously, given the cost and morbidity associated with secondary interventions, the more effective preventative measures will ultimately provide the best path towards optimized PFC function in SZ. And, just as the "vicious negative cycle" can lead patients from poor cognition to poor lifestyle choices to exacerbating extrinsic conditions, it is also anticipated that effective cognitive therapies and PACT strategies will enable patients to make healthier lifestyle choices that promote optimal conditions for PFC function, producing a "positive cycle" to improved quality of life (Figure 1).

CONCLUSION

The PFC plays a critical role in orchestrating neurocognitive processes that are necessary for everyday functioning. Developmental aberrations in the PFC are implicated in the genesis of neurocognitive deficits in SZ; these neurocognitive deficits in turn contribute strongly to the disability burden of this illness. The complex neurochemical environment of PFC poses challenges as well as opportunities for developing pro-cognitive interventions. Sensitive instruments have been developed to systematically assess such interventions, and new strategies for pro-cognitive interventions in SZ have already shown modest yet significant neurocognitive and functional gains. We discuss specific intrinsic and extrinsic factors that may interfere with PFC functioning and thus limit the gains from pro-cognitive intervention, and outline strategies to identify and modify these factors, and thereby optimize PFC functioning and benefits of pro-cognitive interventions. The best strategy for optimizing PFC function, and hence quality of life in SZ patients, involves an integration of what we know about the molecular and cellular biology of this disorder with evidence-based and commonsense approaches to promoting psychological and medical health. This integrative approach to SZ treatment requires continued investment at the levels of basic research and clinical practice models, but its results will be both cost-effective and empowering to patients and families with this disorder.

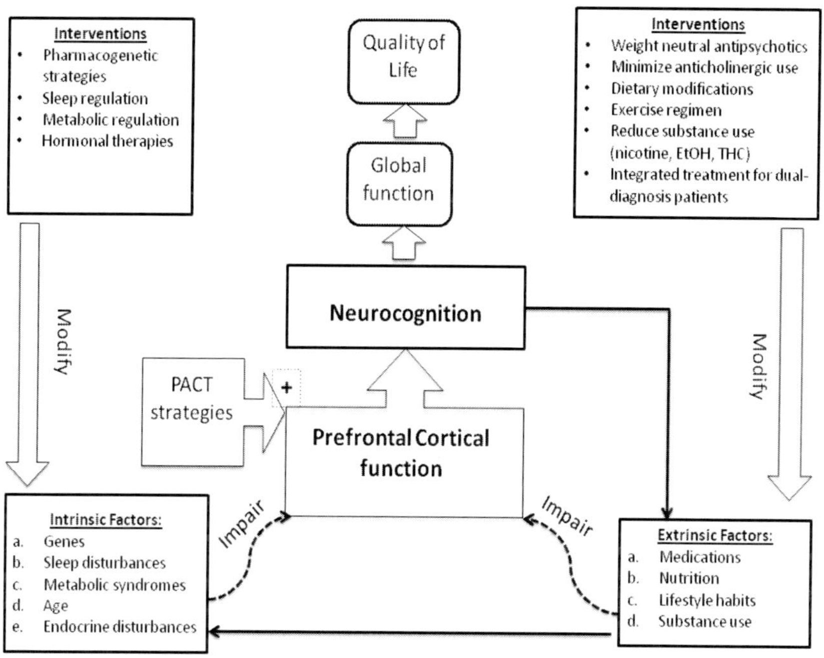

Figure 1. A schematic representation of the "intrinsic" and "extrinsic" factors, impairing prefrontal cortical function, and interventions to modify these factors to optimize prefrontal cortical functioning and thereby improve neurocognition, global function and quality of life. The "solid black line with arrow" indicates "strong influence" and the "+" symbol indicates "positive effect."

ACKNOWLEDGMENTS

Supported by the VISN-22 MIRECC, VA HealthCare System, San Diego, CA, and NIMH Awards MH93453, MH59803 and MH94320. Dr. Swerdlow serves as a Consultant to Neurocrine, Inc.

References

Abi-Saab WM, D'Souza DC, Moghaddam B, Krystal JH (1998) The NMDA antagonist model for schizophrenia: Promise and pitfalls. *Pharmacopsychiatry*, 31 (Suppl. 2), pp. 104–109.

Abernathy K, Chandler LJ, Woodward JJ (2010) Alcohol and the prefrontal cortex. *Int Rev Neurobiol* 91:289-320. doi: 10.1016/S0074-7742(10)91009-X.

Acosta JI, Hiroi R, Camp BW, Talboom JS, Bimonte-Nelson HA (2013) An update on the cognitive impact of clinically-used hormone therapies in the female rat: Models, mazes, and mechanisms. *Brain Res* doi:pii: S0006-8993(13)00065-6. 10.1016/j.brainres.2013.01.016.

AhnAllen CG, Nestor PG, Shenton ME, McCarley RW, Niznikiewicz MA (2008) Early nicotine withdrawal and transdermal nicotine effects on neurocognitive performance in schizophrenia. *Schizophr Res* 100(1-3): 261-9.

American Diabetes Association, American Psychiatric Association (2004) Consensus development conference on antipsychotic drugs and obesity and diabetes. *Diabetes Care* 27:596-601.

Apud JA, Mattay V, Chen J, Kolachana BS, Callicott JH, Rasetti R, Alce G, Iudicello JE, Akbar N, Egan MF, Goldberg TE, Weinberger DR (2007) Tolcapone improves cognition and cortical information processing in normal human subjects. *Neuropsychopharmacology* 32(5):1011-20.

Arime Y, Kasahara Y, Hall FS, Uhl GR, Sora I (2012) Cortico-subcortical neuromodulation involved in the amelioration of prepulse inhibition deficits in dopamine transporter knockout mice. *Neuropsychopharmacology* 37(11):2522-30. doi: 10.1038/npp.2012.114.

Arnsten AF (2004) Adrenergic targets for the treatment of cognitive deficits in schizophrenia. *Psychopharmacology* (Berl) 174(1):25-31.

Arnsten AF (2011) Prefrontal cortical network connections: key site of vulnerability in stress and schizophrenia. *Int J Dev Neurosci* 29(3):215-23. doi: 10.1016/j.ijdevneu.2011.02.006.

Arseneault L, Cannon MC, Poulton R, et al (2002) Cannabis use in adolescence and risk for adult psychosis: longitudinal prospective study. *BMJ*, 325, 1212– 1213.

Atzori G, Lemmonds CA, Kotler ML, Durcan MJ, Boyle J (2008) Efficacy of a nicotine (4 mg)-containing lozenge on the cognitive impairment of nicotine withdrawal. *J Clin Psychopharmacol* 28(6): 667-74.

Averbeck BB, Bobin T, Evans S, Shergill SS (2012) Emotion recognition and oxytocin in patients with schizophrenia. *Psychol Med*; 42:259 – 266.

Awad AG, Voruganti LN (2004) Impact of atypical antipsychotics on quality of life in patients with schizophrenia. *CNS Drugs* 18(13):877-93. Review.

Barbas H, Pandya D (1991) In: Levin HS, Eisenberg HM and Benton AL (eds), *Frontal Lobe Function and Dysfunction*. Oxford Univ. Press, New York, pp 35–58.

Barch DM (2003) Working memory and prefrontal cortex dysfunction: specificity to schizophrenia compared with major depression. *Biol Psychiatry* 53:376–384.

Barch DM (2005) Review: The cognitive neuroscience of schizophrenia. *Annu Rev Clin Psychol.* 1:321-53.

Barch DM, Carter CS (2005) Amphetamine improves cognitive function in medicated individuals with schizophrenia and in healthy volunteers. *Schizophr Res* 77(1):43-58.

Barr RS, Culhane MA, Jubelt LE, Mufti RS, Dyer MA, Weiss AP, Deckersbach T, Kelly JF, Freudenreich O, Goff DC, Evins AE (2008) The effects of transdermal nicotine on cognition in nonsmokers with schizophrenia and nonpsychiatric controls. *Neuropsychopharmacology*; 33(3): 480-90.

Bell MD, Zito W, Greig T, Wexler BE (2008) Neurocognitive enhancement therapy with vocational services: work outcomes at two-year follow-up. *Schizophr Res.* 105(1-3):18-29. doi: 10.1016/j.schres.2008.06.026.

Bell SL, Taylor RC, Singleton EG, Henningfield JE, Heishman SJ (2002) Smoking after nicotine deprivation enhances cognitive performance and decreases tobacco craving in drug abusers. *Nicotine Tob Res* 4(1): 3-4.

Bobo WV, Woodward ND, Sim MY, Jayathilake K, Meltzer HY (2011) The effect of adjunctive armodafinil on cognitive performance and psychopathology in antipsychotic-treated patients with schizophrenia/ schizoaffective disorder: a randomized, double-blind, placebo-controlled trial. *Schizophr Res* 130(1-3):106-13. doi: 10.1016/ j.schres.2011.05.015.

Bou Khalil R, Richa S (2011) Thyroid adverse effects of psychotropic drugs: a review. *Clin Neuropharmacol* 34(6):248-55. doi:10.1097/ WNF.0b013e31823429a7. Review.

Bracy O (1995) CogRcHab Software. Indianapolis, IN: *Psychol. Softw. Serv.*

Bromundt V, Köster M, Georgiev-Kill A, Opwis K, Wirz-Justice A, Stoppe G, Cajochen C (2011) Sleep-wake cycles and cognitive functioning in schizophrenia. *Br J Psychiatry* 198(4):269-76. doi: 10.1192/ bjp.bp.110.078022.

Bromel T, Blum WF, Ziegler A, Schulz E, Bender M, Fleischhaker C (1998). Serum leptin levels increase rapidly after initiation of clozapine therapy.*Mol Psychiatry* 3: 76–80.

Brozoski TJ, Brown R, Rosvold HE, Goldman PS (1979) Cognitive deficit caused by regional depletion of dopamine in the prefrontal cortex of rhesus monkeys. *Science* 205: 929-31.

Bruder TE, Keilp JG, Xu H, et al. (2005) Catechol-O-methyltransferase (COMT) genotypes and working memory: associations with differing cognitive operations. *Biol Psychiatry* 58: 901–7.

Bowie CR, McGurk SR, Mausbach B, Patterson TL, Harvey PD (2012) Combined cognitive remediation and functional skills training for schizophrenia: effects on cognition, functional competence, and real-world behavior. *Am J Psychiatry* 169(7):710-8. doi: 10.1176/appi.ajp. 2012.11091337. PubMed PMID: 22581070.

Bubser M, Koch M (1994) Prepulse inhibition of the acoustic startle response of rats is reduced by 6-hydroxydopamine lesions of the medial prefrontal cortex. *Psychopharmacology* (Berl) 113(3-4):487-92.

Buchanan RW, Keefe RS, Lieberman JA, et al (2011) A randomized clinical trial of & MK-0777 for the treatment of cognitive impairments in people with schizo-phrenia. *Biol Psychiatry* 69:442–449.

Burdick KE, Lencz T, Funke B, et al. (2006) Genetic variation in DTNBP1 influences general cognitive ability. *Hum Mol Genet* 15: 1563-1568.

Burdick KE, Goldberg TE, Funke B, et al. (2007) DTNBP1 genotype influences cognitive decline in schizophrenia. *Schizophr Res* 89: 169–172.

Buschman TJ, Miller EK (2007) Top-down versus bottom-up control of attention in the prefrontal and posterior parietal cortices. *Science* 315:1860–1862.

Carter CJ, Pycock CJ (1980) Behavioural and biochemical effects of dopamine and noradrenaline depletion within the medial prefrontal cortex of the rat. *Brain Res* 192(1):163-76.

Carter CS, Barch DM (2007) Cognitive neuroscience-based approaches to measuring and improving treatment effects on cognition in schizophrenia: the CNTRICS initiative. *Schizophr Bull* 33(5):1131-7. Epub 2007 Jul 14. Review. PubMed PMID: 17630405; PubMed Central PMCID: PMC2632368.

Carter CS, Barch DM, Buchanan RW, Bullmore E, Krystal JH, Cohen J, Geyer M, Green M, Nuechterlein KH, Robbins T, Silverstein S, Smith EE, Strauss M, Wykes T, Heinssen R (2008) Identifying cognitive mechanisms targeted for treatment development in schizophrenia: an overview of the first meeting of the Cognitive Neuroscience Treatment Research to Improve Cognition in Schizophrenia Initiative. *Biol Psychiatry* 64(1):4-10. doi: 10.1016/j.biopsych.2008.03.020.

Chou HH, Twamley E, Swerdlow NR (2012) Towards medication-enhancement of cognitive interventions in schizophrenia. *Handb Exp Pharmacol* (213):81-111. doi: 10.1007/978-3-642-25758-2_4. Review.

Chou HH, Talledo JA, Lamb SN, Thompson WK, Swerdlow NR (2013) Amphetamine effects on MATRICS Consensus Cognitive Battery performance in healthy adults. *Psychopharmacology* (Berl) Jan 12. [Epub ahead of print] PubMed PMID: 23314393.

Cohen JD, Servan-Schreiber D (1992) Context, cortex, and dopamine: A connectionist approach to behavior and biology in schizophrenia. *Psychol. Rev*. 99, 45–77.

Cole MW, Anticevic A, Repovs G, Barch D (2011) Variable global dysconnectivity and individual differences in schizophrenia. *Biol Psychiatry* 70(1):43-50. doi: 10.1016/j.biopsych.2011.02.010. Epub 2011 Apr 15.

Coull JT (1994) Pharmacological manipulations of the a-2 noradrenergic system: effects on cognition. *Drugs Aging* 5:116–126.

Coyle JT (1996) The glutamatergic dysfunction hypothesis for schizophrenia. *Harv. Rev. Psychiatry*, 3, pp. 241–253.

Cramer SC, Sur M, Dobkin BH, O'Brien C, Sanger TD, et al (2011) Harnessing neuroplasticity for clinical applications. *Brain* 134:1591–609.

Creese I, Burt DR, Snyder SH. Dopamine receptor binding predicts clinical and pharmacological potencies of antischizophrenic drugs. *Science* 192:481-483, 1976. PMID: 3854

Das C, Mendez G, Jagasia S, Labbate LA (2012) Second-generation antipsychotic use in schizophrenia and associated weight gain: a critical review and meta-analysis of behavioral and pharmacologic treatments. *Ann Clin Psychiatry* 24(3):225-39. Review. PubMed PMID: 22860242.

Dawson N, Thompson RJ, McVie A, Thomson DM, Morris BJ, Pratt JA (2012) Modafinil reverses phencyclidine-induced deficits in cognitive flexibility, cerebral metabolism, and functional brain connectivity. *Schizophr Bull* 38(3):457-74. doi: 10.1093/schbul/sbq090.

de Lange FP, Koers A, Kalkman JS, Bleijenberg G, Hagoort P, van der Meer JW, Toni I (2008) Increase in prefrontal cortical volume following cognitive behavioural therapy in patients with chronic fatigue syndrome. *Brain* 131:2172–2180. doi:10.1093/brain de Leon J, Diaz FJ (2005) A meta-analysis of worldwide studies demonstrates an association between schizophrenia and tobacco smoking behaviors. *Schizophr Res* 76(2-3):135-57. PubMed PMID: 15949648.

de Lucena D, Fernandes BS, Berk M, Dodd S, Medeiros DW, Pedrini M, Kunz M, Gomes FA, Giglio LF, Lobato MI, Belmonte-de-Abreu PS, Gama CS (2009) Improvement of negative and positive symptoms in treatment-refractory schizophrenia: a double-blind, randomized, placebo-controlled trial with memantine as add-on therapy to clozapine. *J Clin Psychiatry* 70(10):1416-23. doi: 10.4088/JCP.08m04935gry.

Desmarais JE, Beauclair L, Margolese HC (2012) Anticholinergics in the era of atypical antipsychotics: short-term or long-term treatment? *J Psychopharmacol* 26(9):1167-74. doi: 10.1177/0269881112447988.

Deutch AY (1992) The regulation of subcortical dopamine systems by the prefrontal cortex: interactions of central dopamine systems and the pathogenesis of schizophrenia. *J Neural Transm Suppl* 36:61-89. Review.

Deutsch SI, Rosse RB, Schwartz BL, Mastropaolo J (2001) A revised excitotoxic hypothesis of schizophrenia: therapeutic implications. *Clin Neuropharmacol* 24(1):43-9. Review.

Dickinson D, Gold JM, Dickerson FB, Medoff D, Dixon LB (2008) Evidence of exacerbated cognitive deficits in schizophrenia patients with comorbid diabetes. *Psychosomatics* 49(2):123-31. doi: 10.1176/appi.psy.49.2.123.

Dohanich GP (2002) Gonadal steroids, learning and memory. In: Pfaff DW, Arnold AP, Etgen AM, Fahrbach SE, Rubin RI (Eds.) *Hormones, brain and behavior*. Academic Press, San Diego pp. 265–327.

Domes G, Heinrichs M, Michel A, et al. (2007) Oxytocin improves 'mind-reading' in humans. *Biol Psychiatry* 61:731 – 733.

Dreher JC, Koch P, Kohn P, Apud J, Weinberger DR, Berman KF (2012) Common and differential pathophysiological features accompany comparable cognitive impairments in medication-free patients with schizophrenia and in healthy aging subjects. *Biol Psychiatry* 71(10):890-7. doi: 10.1016/j.biopsych.2012.01.002.

Driscoll I, Martin B, An Y, Maudsley S, Ferrucci L, Mattson MP, Resnick SM (2012) Plasma BDNF is associated with age-related white matter atrophy but not with cognitive function in older, non-demented adults. *PLoS One*, 7 (4), p. e35217

D'Souza DC, Perry E, MacDougall L, Ammerman Y, Cooper T, Wu YT, Braley G,Gueorguieva R, Krystal JH (2004) The psychotomimetic effects of intravenous delta-9-tetrahydrocannabinol in healthy individuals: implications for psychosis. *Neuropsychopharmacology* 29(8):1558-72.

D'Souza DC, Abi-Saab WM, Madonick S, Forselius-Bielen K, Doersch A, Braley G, Gueorguieva R, Cooper TB, Krystal JH (2005) Delta-9-tetrahydrocannabinol effects in schizophrenia: implications for cognition, psychosis, and addiction. *Biol Psychiatry* 57(6):594-608.

Eack SM, Hogarty GE, Greenwald DP, Hogarty SS, Keshavan MS (2006) Cognitive enhancement therapy improves emotional intelligence in early course schizophrenia: preliminary effects. *Schizophr Res* 89(1-3):308-11.

Eack SM, Hogarty GE, Cho RY, et al. (2010) Neuroprotective effects of cognitive enhancement therapy against gray matter loss in early schizophrenia: results from a 2-year randomized controlled trial. *Arch Gen Psychiatry* 67:674 – 682.

Egan MF, Goldberg TE, Kolachana BS, Callicott JH, Mazzanti CM, Straub RE, Goldman D, Weinberger DR (2001) Effect of COMT Val108/158 Met genotype on frontal lobe function and risk for schizophrenia. *Proc Natl Acad Sci U S A* 98:6917–6922.

Eggan SM, Hashimoto T, Lewis DA (2008) Reduced cortical cannabinoid 1 receptor messenger RNA and protein expression in schizophrenia. *Arch Gen Psychiatry* 65(7):772-84. doi: 10.1001/archpsyc.65.7.772.

Elman I, Borsook D, Lukas SE (2006) Food intake and reward mechanisms in patients with schizophrenia: implications for metabolic disturbances and treatment with second-generation antipsychotic agents. *Neuropsychopharmacology* 31(10):2091-120. Review

Ellenbroek BA, Budde S, Cools AR (1996) Prepulse inhibition and latent inhibition: the role of dopamine in the medial prefrontal cortex. *Neuroscience* 75(2):535-42.

Elliott R, Sahakian BJ, Matthews K, Bannerjea A, Rimmer J, Robbins TW (1997) Effects of methylphenidate on spatial working memory and planning in healthy young adults. *Psychopharmacology* (Berl) 131: 196-206.

Evans DE, Drobes DJ (2009) Nicotine self-medication of cognitive-attentional processing. *Addict Biol* 14(1): 32-42.

Evins AE, Fitzgerald SM, Wine L, Rosselli R, Goff DC (2000) Placebo-controlled trial of glycine added to clozapine in schizophrenia. *Am. J. Psychiatry* 157, pp. 826–828.

Farreny A, Aguado J, Ochoa S, Huerta-Ramos E, Marsà F, López-Carrilero R, Carral V, Haro JM, Usall J (2012) REPYFLEC cognitive remediation group training in schizophrenia: Looking for an integrative approach. *Schizophr Res* 142(1-3):137-44. doi: 10.1016/j.schres.2012.08.035.

Feifel D, Reza T (1999) Oxytocin modulates psychotomimetic-induced deficits in sensorimotor gating. *Psychopharmacology* (Berl) 141:93 – 98.

Feifel D, Macdonald K, Nguyen A, et al (2010) Adjunctive intranasal oxytocin reduces symptoms in schizophrenia patients. *Biol Psychiatry* 68:678 – 680.

Feifel D, Macdonald K, Cobb P, Minassian A (2012) Adjunctive intranasal oxytocin improves verbal memory in people with schizophrenia. *Schizophr Res* 139:207 – 210.

Fields RB, Van Kammen DP, Peters JL, Rosen J, Van Kammen WB, Nugent A, Stipetic M, Linnoila M (1988) Clonidine improves memory function in schizophrenia independently from change in psychosis. *Schizophr Res* 1:417–423.

Field CD, Galletly C, Anderson D, Walfer P (1997) Computer-aided cognitive rehabilitation: possible application to the attentional deficit of schizophrenia, a report of negative results. *Perceptual and Motor Skills* 85, 995–1002.

Fisher M, Holland C, Merzenich MM, Vinogradov S (2009) Using neuroplasticity-based auditory training to improve verbal memory in schizophrenia. *Am J Psychiatry* 166:805-811.

Fisher M, Holland C, Subramaniam K, Vinogradov S (2010) Neuroplasticity-based cognitive training in schizophrenia: an interim report on the effects 6 months later. *Schizophr Bull* 36:869-879. PMCID: PMC2894606

Flores CM, Rogers SW, Pabreza LA, Wolfe BB, Kellar KJ (1992) A subtype of nicotinic cholinergic receptor in rat brain is composed of alpha 4 and beta 2 subunits and is up-regulated by chronic nicotine treatment. *Mol Pharmacol* 41:31–37.

Fox K (2009) Experience-dependent plasticity mechanisms for neural rehabilitation in somatosensory cortex. *Philos Trans R Soc Lond Series B Biol Sci* 364:369–381. doi:10.1098/rstb.2008.0252

Freedman R, Olincy A, Buchanan RW, Harris JG, Gold JM, Johnson L, Allensworth D, Guzman-Bonilla A, Clement B, Ball MP, Kutnick J, Pender V, Martin LF, Stevens KE, Wagner BD, Zerbe GO, Soti F, Kem WR (2008) Initial phase 2 trial of a nicotinic agonist in schizophrenia. *Am J Psychiatry* 165(8):1040-7. doi: 10.1176/appi.ajp.2008.07071135.

Friedman JI, Adler DN, Temporini HD, Kemether E, Harvey PD, White L, Parrella M, Davis KL (2001) Guanfacine treatment of cognitive impairment in schizophrenia. *Neuropsychopharmacology* 25(3):402-9. PubMed PMID: 11522468.

Friedman JI, Wallenstein S, Moshier E, Parrella M, White L, Bowler S, et al. (2010) The effects of hypertension and body mass index on cognition in schizophrenia. *Am. J. Psychiatry* 167 (10), 1232–1239.

Fujimaki K, Takahashi T, Morinobu S (2012) Association of typical versus atypical antipsychotics with symptoms and quality of life in schizophrenia. *PLoS One7*(5):e37087. doi: 10.1371/journal.pone.0037087.

Fuster JM (1989) *The Prefrontal Cortex*. Raven Press, New York.

Gasbarri A, Tavares MC, Rodrigues RC, Tomaz C, Pompili A (2012) Estrogen, cognitive functions and emotion: an overview on humans, non-human primates and rodents in reproductive years. *Rev Neurosci* doi:pii: /j/revneuro.ahead-of-print/revneuro-2012-0051/revneuro-2012-0051.xml. 10.1515/revneuro-2012-0051.

George MS, Molnar CE, Grenesko EL, Anderson B, Mu Q, Johnson K, Nahas Z, Knable M, Fernandes P, Juncos J, Huang X, Nichols DE, Mailman RB (2007) A single 20 mg dose of dihydrexidine (DAR-0100), a full dopamine D1 agonist, is safe and tolerated in patients with schizophrenia. *Schizophr Res* 93(1-3):42-50.

Ghika J (2008) Paleoneurology: Neurodegenerative diseases are age-related diseases of specific brain regions recently developed by Homo sapiens. *Medical Hypotheses*, 71, pp. 788–801.

Giakoumaki SG, Roussos P, Bitsios P (2008) Improvement of prepulse inhibition and executive function by the COMT inhibitor tolcapone depends on COMT Val158Met polymorphism. *Neuropsychopharmacology* 33(13):3058-68. doi: 10.1038/npp.2008.82.

Goff DC, Leahy L, Berman I, Posever T, Herz L, Leon AC, Johnson SA, Lynch G (2001) A placebo-controlled pilot study of the ampakine CX516 added to clozapine in schizophrenia. *J. Clin. Psychopharmacol* 21, pp. 484–487.

Goff DC, Sullivan LM, McEvoy JP, Meyer JM, Nasrallah HA, Daumit GL, Lamberti S, D'Agostino RB, Stroup TS, Davis S, Lieberman JA (2005) A comparison of ten-year cardiac risk estimates in schizophrenia patients from the CATIE study and matched controls. *Schizophr Res* 80(1):45-53.

Goff DC, Lamberti JS, Leon AC, Green MF, Miller AL, Patel J, Manschreck T, Freudenreich O, Johnson SA (2008a) A placebo-controlled add-on trial of the Ampakine, CX516, for cognitive deficits in schizophrenia. *Neuropsychopharmacology* 33(3):465-72.

Goff DC, Cather C, Gottlieb JD, Evins AE, Walsh J, Raeke L, Otto MW, Schoenfeld D, Green MF (2008b) Once-weekly D-cycloserine effects on negative symptoms and cognition in schizophrenia: an exploratory study. *Schizophr Res* 106(2-3):320-7. doi: 10.1016/j.schres.2008.08.012.

Gold PE (2003) Acetylcholine modulation of neural systems involved in learning and memory. *Neurobiol. Learn. Mem.* 80:194–210.

Goldberg TE, Bigelow LB, Weinberger DR, Daniel DG, Kleinman JE (1991) Cognitive and behavioral effects of the coadministration of dextroamphetamine and haloperidol in schizophrenia. *Am J Psychiatry* 148:78–84

Goldberg TE, Straub RE, Callicott JH, et al. (2006) The G72/G30 gene complex and cognitive abnormalities in schizophrenia. *Neuropsychopharmacology* 31: 2022–2032.

Gothelf D, Falk B, Singer P, Kairi M, Phillip M, Zigel L et al (2002). Weight gain associated with increased food intake and low habitual activity levels in male adolescent schizophrenic inpatients treated with olanzapine. *Am J Psychiatry* 159: 1055–1057.

Gottlieb JD, Cather C, Shanahan M, Creedon T, Macklin EA, Goff DC (2011) D-cycloserine facilitation of cognitive behavioral therapy for delusions in schizophrenia. *Schizophr Res* 131(1-3):69-74. doi: 10.1016/j.schres. 2011.05.029.

Grant KM, LeVan TD, Wells SM, Li M, Stoltenberg SF, Gendelman HE, Carlo G, Bevins RA (2012) Methamphetamine-associated psychosis. *J Neuroimmune Pharmacol* 7(1):113-39. doi: 10.1007/s11481-011-9288-1.

Granholm E, McQuaid JR, McClure FS, Link PC, Perivoliotis D, Gottlieb JD, Patterson TL, Jeste DV (2007) Randomized controlled trial of cognitive behavioral social skills training for older people with schizophrenia: 12-month follow-up. *J Clin Psychiatry* 68(5):730-7.

Gray JA, Roth BL (2007) Molecular targets for treating cognitive dysfunction in schizophrenia. *Schizophr Bull* 33(5):1100-19. Review.

Green MF, Nuechterlein KH, Gold JM, Barch DM, Cohen J, Essock S, Fenton WS, Frese F, Goldberg TE, Heaton RK, Keefe RS, Kern RS, Kraemer H, Stover E, Weinberger DR, Zalcman S, Marder SR (2004a) Approaching a consensus cognitive battery for clinical trials in schizophrenia: the NIMH-MATRICS conference to select cognitive domains and test criteria. *Biol Psychiatry* 56(5):301-7. Review. PubMed PMID: 15336511.

Green MF, Kern RS, Heaton RK (2004b) Longitudinal studies of cognition and functional outcome in schizophrenia: implications for MATRICS. *Schizophr Res* 72:41–51. doi:10.1016/j.schres.2004.09.009

Green B, Young R, Kavanagh D (2005) Cannabis use and misuse prevalence among people with psychosis. *BJP* 187:306-313; doi:10.1192/bjp.187.4.306

Grillon ML, Oppenheim C, Varoquaux G, Charbonneau F, Devauchelle AD, Krebs MO, Bayle F, Thirion B, Huron C (2012) Hyperfrontality and hypoconnectivity during refreshing in schizophrenia. *Psychiatry Res pii:* S0925-4927(12)00214-4. doi: 10.1016/j.pscychresns.2012.09.001.

Gruber AJ, Calhoon GG, Shusterman I, Schoenbaum G, Roesch MR, O'Donnell P (2010) More is less: a disinhibited prefrontal cortex impairs cognitive flexibility. *J Neurosci* 30(50):17102-10. doi: 10.1523/JNEUROSCI.4623-10.2010.

Grynszpan O, Perbal S, Pelissolo A, Fossati P, Jouvent R, Dubal S, Perez-Diaz F (2011) Efficacy and specificity of computer-assisted cognitive remediation in schizophrenia: a meta-analytical study. *Psychol Med* 41(1):163-73. doi: 10.1017/S0033291710000607.

Gupta A, Craig TK (2009) Diet, smoking and cardiovascular risk in schizophrenia in high and low care supported housing. *Epidemiol Psichiatr Soc* 18(3):200-7.

Hall H, Sedvall G, Magnusson O, Kopp J, Halldin C, Farde L. Distribution of D1- and D2-dopamine receptors, and dopamine and its metabolites in the human brain. *Neuropsychopharmacology* 11:245–256, 1994. PMID: 7531978.

Hallmayer JF, Kalaydjieva L, Badcock J, et al. (2005) Genetic evidence for a distinct subtype of schizophrenia characterized by pervasive cognitive deficit. *Am J Hum Genet* 77: 468–476.

Hamidovic A, Dlugos A, Palmer AA, de Wit H (2010) Catechol-Omethyltransferase val158met genotype modulates sustained attention in both the drug-free state and in response to amphetamine. *Psychiatr Genet* 20:85–92. PMCID: PMC2875066

Hampson RE, Rogers G, Lynch G, Deadwyler SA (1998a) Facilitative effects of the ampakine CX516 on short-term memory in rats: Correlations with hippocampal neuronal activity. *J. Neurosci* 18, pp. 2748–2763.

Hampson RE, Rogers G, Lynch G, Deadwyler SA (1998b) Facilitative effects of the ampakine CX516 on short-term memory in rats: Enhancement of delayed-nonmatch-to-sample performance. *J. Neurosci* 18, pp. 2740–2747.

Harrison PJ, Lyon L, Sartorius LJ, et al. (2008) The group II metabotropic glutamate receptor 3 (mGluR3, mGlu3, GRM3): expression, function and involvement in schizophrenia. *J Psychopharmacol* 22: 308–322.

Heal DJ, Gosden J, Jackson HC, Cheetham SC, Smith SL (2012) Metabolic consequences of antipsychotic therapy: preclinical and clinical perspectives on diabetes, diabetic ketoacidosis, and obesity. *Handb Exp Pharmacol* (212):135-64. doi: 10.1007/978-3-642-25761-2_6.

Henderson DC, Borba CP, Daley TB, Boxill R, Nguyen DD, Culhane MA, Louie P, Cather C, Eden Evins A, Freudenreich O, Taber SM, Goff DC (2006) Dietary intake profile of patients with schizophrenia. *Ann Clin Psychiatry* 18(2):99-105. PubMed PMID: 16754415.

Heresco-Levy U, Javitt DC, Ermilov M, Mordel C, Silipo G, Lichtenstein M (1999) Efficacy of high-dose glycine in the treatment of enduring negative symptoms of schizophrenia *Arch. Gen. Psychiatry* 56, pp. 29–36.

Heresco-Levy U, Ermilov M, Lichtenberg P, Bar G, Javitt DC (2004) High-dose glycine added to olanzapine and risperidone for the treatment of schizophrenia. *Biol. Psychiatry* 55, pp. 165–171.

Heresco-Levy U, Javitt DC, Ebstein R, Vass A, Lichtenberg P, Bar G, Catinari S, Ermilov M (2005) D-serine efficacy as add-on pharmacotherapy to risperidone and olanzapine for treatment-refractory schizophrenia. *Biol. Psychiatry* 57, pp. 577–585.

Hill JO, Bessesen D (2003) What to do about the metabolic syndrome? *Arch Intern Med* 163(4):395-7.

Honea R, Crow TJ, Passingham D, Mackay CE (2005) Regional deficits in brain volume in schizophrenia: a meta-analysis of voxel-based morphometry studies. *Am J Psychiatry* 162(12):2233-45. Review.

Horisawa T, Nishikawa H, Toma S, Ikeda A, Horiguchi M, Ono M, Ishiyama T, Taiji M (2013) The role of 5-HT(7) receptor antagonism in the amelioration of MK-801-induced learning and memory deficits by the novel atypical antipsychotic drug lurasidone. *Behav Brain Res* pii: S0166-4328(13)00045-4. doi: 10.1016/j.bbr.2013.01.026.

Hughes JR, Hatsukami DK, Mitchell JE, Dahlgren LA (1986) Prevalence of smoking among psychiatric outpatients. *Am J Psychiatry* 143(8):993-7.

Hughes JR, Helzer JE, Lindberg SA (2006) Prevalence of DSM/ICD-defined nicotine dependence. *Drug Alcohol Depend* 85(2):91-102.

Hunault CC, Mensinga TT, B^cker KB, Schipper CM, Kruidenier M, Leenders ME, de Vries I, Meulenbelt J (2009) Cognitive and psychomotor effects in males after smoking acombination of tobacco and cannabis containing up to 69 mg delta-9 tetrahydrocannabinol (THC). *Psychopharmacology* (Berl) 204(1):85-94. doi: 10.1007/s00213-008-1440-0.

Ichioka S, Terao T, Hoaki N, Matsushita T, Hoaki T (2012) Triiodothyronine may be possibly associated with better cognitive function and less extrapyramidal symptoms in chronic schizophrenia. Prog Neuropsychopharmacol *Biol Psychiatry* 39(1):170-4. doi: 10.1016/j.pnpbp.2012.06.008.

Iosifescu DV, Gilmer WS, Fan A, Gonenc A, Moore C, Randolph C, Rapaport MH, Peters A, Deckersbach T, Nierenberg AA (2012) Memantine for Cognitive Dysfunction in Bipolar Disorder and Correlation with Hippocampal Neuronal Viability. *Biological Psychiatry* 71(8):1S-106S *Supplement.*

Ingvar M, Ambros-Ingerson J, Davis M, Granger R, Kessler M, Rogers GA, Schehr RS, Lynch G (1997) Enhancement by an ampakine of memory encoding in humans. *Exp. Neurol* 146, pp. 553–559.

Jaffe F, Markov D, Doghramji K (2006) Sleep-disordered breathing: in depression and schizophrenia. *Psychiatry* (Edgmont) 3(7):62-8.

Jakala P, Riekkinen M, Sirvio J, Koivisto E, Kejonen K, Vanhanen M, Riekkinen PJ (1999a) Guanfacine, but not clonidine, improves planning and working memory performance in humans. *Neuropsychopharmacology* 20:460–470.

Jakala P, Sirvio J, Riekkinen M, Koivisto E, Kejonen K, Vanhanen M, Riekkinen PJ (1999b) Guanfacine and clonidine, alpha-2 agonists, improve paired associates learning, but not delayed matching to sample, in humans. *Neuropsychopharmacology* 20:119–130.

Javitt DC (1987) Negative schizophrenic symptomatology and the PCP (phencyclidine) model of schizophrenia. *Hillside J. Clin. Psychiatry* 9, pp. 12–35.

Javitt DC, Silipo G, Cienfuegos A, Shelley AM, Bark N, Park M, Lindenmayer JP, Suckow R, Zukin SR (2001) Adjunctive high-dose glycine in the treatment of schizophrenia. *Int. J. Neuropsychopharmacol* 4, pp. 385–392.

Javitt DC, Hashim A, Sershen H (2005) Modulation of striatal dopamine release by glycine transport inhibitors. *Neuropsychopharmacology* 30, pp. 649–656.

Javitt DC (2007) Glutamate and schizophrenia: phencyclidine, N-methyl-D-aspartate receptors, and dopamine-glutamate interactions. *Int Rev Neurobiol* 78:69-108. Review.

Jentsch JD, Roth RH (1999) The neuropsychopharmacology of phencyclidine: From NMDA receptor hypofunction to the dopamine hypothesis of schizophrenia. *Neuropsychopharmacology* 20, pp. 201–225.

Kane JM, Barrett EJ, Casey DE, Correll CU, Gelenberg AJ, Klein S et al(2004). Metabolic effects of treatment with atypical antipsychotics. *J Clin Psychiatry* 65: 1447–1455.

Kane JM, D'Souza DC, Patkar AA, Youakim JM, Tiller JM, Yang R, Keefe RS (2010) Armodafinil as adjunctive therapy in adults with cognitive deficits associated with schizophrenia: a 4-week, double-blind, placebo-controlled study. *J Clin Psychiatry* 71(11):1475-81. doi: 10.4088/JCP.09m05950gry.

Kantrowitz JT, Malhotra AK, Cornblatt B, Silipo G, Balla A, Suckow RF, D'Souza C, Saksa J, Woods SW, Javitt DC (2010) High dose D-serine in the treatment of schizophrenia. *Schizophr Res* 121(1-3):125-30. doi: 10.1016/j.schres.2010.05.012.

Keedy SK, Ebens CL, Keshavan MS, Sweeney JA (2006) Functional magnetic resonance imaging studies of eye movements in first episode schizophrenia: smooth pursuit, visually guided saccades and the oculomotor delayed response task. *Psychiatry Res* 146:199–211.

Keefe RS, Perkins DO, Gu H, Zipursky RB, Christensen BK, Lieberman JA (2006a) A longitudinal study of neurocognitive function in individuals at-risk for psychosis. *Schizophr Res.* 88(1-3):26-35.

Keefe RS, Bilder RM, Harvey PD, Davis SM, Palmer BW, Gold JM, Meltzer HY, Green MF, Miller DD, Canive JM, Adler LW, Manschreck TC, Swartz M, Rosenheck R, Perkins DO, Walker TM, Stroup TS, McEvoy JP, Lieberman JA (2006b) Baseline neurocognitive deficits in the CATIE schizophrenia trial. *Neuropsychopharmacology* 31(9):2033-46.

Kelleher JP, Centorrino F, Huxley NA, Bates JA, Drake JK, Egli S, Baldessarini RJ (2012) Pilot randomized, controlled trial of pramipexole to augment antipsychotic treatment. Eur *Neuropsychopharmacol* 22(6):415-8. doi: 10.1016/j.euroneuro.2011.10.002.

Keller TA, Just MA (2009) Altering cortical connectivity: remediation-induced changes in the white matter of poor readers. *Neuron* 64:624–631. doi:10.1016/j.neuron.2009.10.018.

Kern RS, Green MF, Nuechterlein KH, Deng BH (2004) NIMH-MATRICS survey on assessment of neurocognition in schizophrenia. *Schizophr Res.* 72(1):11-9.

Kern RS, Nuechterlein KH, Green MF, Baade LE, Fenton WS, Gold JM, Keefe RS, Mesholam-Gately R, Mintz J, Seidman LJ, Stover E, Marder

SR (2008) The MATRICS Consensus Cognitive Battery, part 2: co-norming and standardization. *Am J Psychiatry* 165(2):214-20. doi: 10.1176/appi.ajp.2007.07010043.

Keshavan MS, Montrose DM, Miewald JM, Jindal RD (2011) Sleep correlates of cognition in early course psychotic disorders. *Schizophr Res* 131(1-3):231-4. doi: 10.1016/j.schres.2011.05.027.

Kidd PM (2007) Omega-3 DHA and EPA for cognition, behavior, and mood: clinical findings and structural-functional synergies with cell membrane phospholipids. *Altern Med Rev* 12(3):207-27.

Killgore WD (2010) Effects of sleep deprivation on cognition. *Prog Brain Res* 185:105-29. doi: 10.1016/B978-0-444-53702-7.00007-5.

Kimberg DY, D'Esposito M, Farah MJ (1997) Effects of bromocriptine on human subjects depends on working memory capacity. *Neuroreport* 8: 3581-3585.

Kinon BJ, Kaiser CJ, Ahmed S, Rotelli MD, Kollack-Walker S (2005). Association between early and rapid weight gain and change in weight over one year of olanzapine therapy in patients with schizophrenia and related disorders. *J Clin Psychopharmacol* 25: 255–258.

Kircher T, Krug A, Markov V, et al. (2009) Genetic variation in the schizophrenia-risk gene neuregulin 1 correlates with brain activation and impaired speech production in a verbal fluency task in healthy individuals. *Hum Brain Mapp* 30: 3406–3416.

Kirrane RM, Mitropoulou V, Nunn M, New AS, Harvey PD, Schopick F, Silverman J, Siever LJ (2000) Effects of amphetamine on visuospatial working memory performance in schizophrenia spectrum personality disorder. *Neuropsychopharmacology* 22(1):14-8.

Kluwe-Schiavon B, Sanvicente-Vieira B, Kristensen CH, Grassi-Oliveira R (2013) Executive functions rehabilitation for schizophrenia: a critical systematic review. *J Psychiatr Res* 47(1):91-104. doi: 10.1016/ j.jpsychires.2012.10.001.

Kontis D, Huddy V, Reeder C, Landau S, Wykes T (2013) Effects of Age and Cognitive Reserve on Cognitive Remediation Therapy Outcome in Patients With Schizophrenia. *Am J Geriatr Psychiatry* 21(3):218-30. doi: 10.1016/j.jagp.2012.12.013.

Korosi A, Baram TZ (2009) The pathways from mother's love to baby's future. *Front Behav Neurosci* 3:27. doi:10.3389/neuro.08.027.2009.

Kosfeld M, Heinrichs M, Zak PJ, et al (2005) Oxytocin increases trust in humans. *Nature* 435:673 – 676.

Knight RT, Grabowecky MF, Scabini D (1995) Role of human prefrontal cortex in attention control. *Adv Neurol* 66:21–34.

Krug A, Markov V, Krach S, et al. (2010) The effect of Neuregulin 1 on neural correlates of episodic memory encoding and retrieval. *Neuro-image* 53: 985–991.

Krystal JH, Abi- Saab W, Perry E, D'Souza DC, Liu N, Gueorguieva R, McDougall L, Hunsberger T, Belger A, Levine L, Breier A (2005) Preliminary evidence of attenuation of the disruptive effects of the NMDA glutamate receptor antagonist, ketamine, on working memory by pretreatment with the group II metabotropic glutamate receptor agonist, LY354740, in healthy human subjects. *Psychopharmacology* (Berl.) 179 (1), pp. 303–309.

Kuepper R, Skinbjerg M, Abi-Dargham A (2012) The dopamine dysfunction in schizophrenia revisited: new insights into topography and course. *Handb Exp Pharmacol* (212):1-26. PMID: 23129326 "PMC Journal – In Process"

Kurlan R (2003) Tourette's syndrome: are stimulants safe? *Curr Neurol Neurosci Rep* 3:285-288.

Lebois EP, Bridges TM, Lewis LM, Dawson ES, Kane AS, Xiang Z, Jadhav SB, Yin H, Kennedy JP, Meiler J, Niswender CM, Jones CK, Conn PJ, Weaver CD, Lindsley CW (2010) Discovery and characterization of novel subtype-selective allosteric agonists for the investigation of M1 receptor function in the central nervous system. *ACS Chem Neurosci* 1:104–121.

Lee D, Rushworth MF, Walton ME, Watanabe M, Sakagami M (2007) Functional specialization of the primate frontal cortex during decision making. *J Neurosci* 27:8170–8173.

Lee JG, Lee SW, Lee BJ, Park SW, Kim GM, Kim YH (2012) Adjunctive memantine therapy for cognitive impairment in chronic schizophrenia: a placebo-controlled pilot study. *Psychiatry Investig.* Jun;9(2):166-73. doi: 10.4306/pi.2012.9.2.166.

Lee PR, Brady DL, Shapiro RA, et al (2005) Social interaction deficits caused by chronic phencyclidine administration are reversed by oxytocin. *Neuropsycho- pharmacology* 30:1883 – 1894.

Leonard S, Adler LE, Benhammou K, Berger R, Breese CR, Drebing C, Gault J, Lee MJ, Logel J, Olincy A, Ross RG, Stevens K, Sullivan B, Vianzon R, Virnich DE, Waldo M, Walton K, Freedman R (2001) Smoking and mental illness. *Pharmacol Biochem Behav* 70(4):561-70. Review.

Lenroot RK, Giedd JN (2006) Brain development in children and adolescents: Insights from anatomical magnetic resonance imaging. *Neuroscience and Biobehavioral Reviews,* 30, pp. 718–729.

Leucht S, Arbter D, Engel RR, Kissling W, Davis JM (2009) How effective are second-generation antipsychotic drugs? A meta-analysis of placebo-controlled trials. *Mol Psychiatry* 14:429–447.

Levin ED, McClernon FJ, Rezvani AH (2006) Nicotinic effects on cognitive function: behavioral characterization, pharmacological specification, and anatomic localization. *Psychopharmacology* (Berl.) 184:523–539.

Lewis DA, Hashimoto T, Volk DW (2005) Cortical inhibitory neurons and schizo- phrenia. *Nat Rev Neurosci* 6:312–324.

Lewis DA, Cho RY, Carter CS, et al (2008) Subunit-selective modulation of GABAtype A receptor neurotransmission and cognition in schizophrenia. *Am JPsychiatry* 165:1585–1593.

Lieberman JA, Stroup TS, McEvoy JP, Swartz MS, Rosenheck RA, Perkins DO, Keefe RS, Davis SM, Davis CE, Lebowitz BD, Severe J, Hsiao JK (2005) Effectiveness of antipsychotic drugs in patients with chronic schizophrenia. *N Engl J Med* 353:1209–1223.

Lindenmayer JP, Khan A (2011) Galantamine augmentation of long-acting injectable risperidone for cognitive impairments in chronic schizophrenia. *Schizophr Res*;125:267-77.

Lindenmayer JP, Khan A, Kaushik S, Thanju A, Praveen R, Hoffman L, Cherath L, Valdez G, Wance D (2012) *Schizophr Res* 142(1-3):171-6. doi: 10.1016/j.schres.2012.09.019.

Lorrain DS, Baccei CS, Bristow LJ, Anderson JJ, Varney MA (2003) Effects of ketamine and N-methyl-D-aspartate on glutamate and dopamine release in the rat prefrontal cortex: Modulation by a group II selective metabotropic glutamate receptor agonist LY379268. *Neuroscience* 117, pp. 697–706.

Lotta T, Vidgren J, Tilgmann C, Ulmanen I, Melén K, Julkunen I, Taskinen J (1995) Kinetics of human soluble and membrane-bound catechol O-methyltransferase: a revised mechanism and description of the thermolabile variant of the enzyme. *Biochemistry* 34(13):4202-10.

Lovio R, Halttunen A, Lyytinen H, Näätänen R, Kujala T (2012) Reading skill and neural processing accuracy improvement after a 3-hour intervention in preschoolers with difficulties in reading-related skills. *Brain Res* 1448:42-55.

Luine VN (2008) Sex steroids and cognitive function. *J Neuroendocrinol* 20 pp. 866–872.

Luine V, Frankfurt M (2012) Interactions between estradiol, BDNF and dendritic spines in promoting memory. *Neuroscience*. pii: S0306-4522(12)01027-5. doi: 10.1016/j.neuroscience.2012.10.019.

Ma L, Seager MA, Wittmann M, Jacobson M, Bickel D, Burno M, Jones K, Graufelds VK, Xu G, Pearson M, McCampbell A, Gaspar R, Shughrue P, Danziger A, Regan C, Flick R, Pascarella D, Garson S, Doran S, Kreatsoulas C, Veng L, Lindsley CW, Shipe W, Kuduk S, Sur C, Kinney G, Seabrook GR, Ray WJ (2009) Selective activation of the M1 muscarinic acetylcholine receptor achieved by allosteric potentiation. *Proc Natl Acad Sci U S A* 106:15950–15955.

Marenco S, Egan MF, Goldberg TE, Knable MB, McClure RK, Winterer G, Weinberger DR (2002) Preliminary experience with an ampakine (CX516) as a single agent for the treatment of schizophrenia: A case series. *Schizophr. Res.*, 57, pp. 221–226.

Marker KR (2001) *COGPACK 6.0*. Markersoftware, Ladenburg.

Markham JA, Mullins SE, Koenig JI(2012)Peri-adolescent maturation of the prefrontal cortex is sex-specific and disrupted by prenatal stress. *J Comp Neurol.* Nov 21. doi: 10.1002/cne.23262.

Martin LF, Kem WR, Freedman R (2004) Alpha-7 nicotinic receptor agonists: potential new candidates for the treatment of schizophrenia. *Psychopharmacology* (Berl) 174(1):54-64.

Mattay VS, Goldberg TE, Fera F, et al. (2003) Catechol O-methyltrans- ferase val158-met genotype and individual variation in the brain response to amphetamine. *Proc Natl Acad Sci U S A* 100: 6186–6191.

McCann UD, Szabo Z, Vranesic M, Palermo M, Mathews WB, Ravert HT, Dannals RF, Ricaurte GA (2008) Positron emission tomographic studies of brain dopamine and serotonin transporters in abstinent (+/-)3,4-methylenedioxymethamphetamine ("ecstasy") users: relationship to cognitive performance. *Psychopharmacology* (Berl) 200(3):439-50. doi: 10.1007/s00213-008-1218-4.

McCloughen A (2003) The association between schizophrenia and cigarette smoking: a review of the literature and implications for mental health nursing practice. *Int J Ment Health Nurs* 12(2):119-29. PubMed PMID: 12956023.

McClure MM, Harvey PD, Goodman M, Triebwasser J, New A, Koenigsberg HW, Sprung LJ, Flory JD, Siever LJ (2010) Pergolide treatment of cognitive deficits associated with schizotypal personality disorder: continued evidence of the importance of the dopamine system in the schizophrenia spectrum. *Neuropsychopharmacology* 35(6):1356-62. doi: 10.1038/npp.2010.5.

McCreadie RG; Scottish Schizophrenia Lifestyle Group (2003) Diet, smoking and cardiovascular risk in people with schizophrenia: descriptive study. *Br J Psychiatry* 183:534-9.

McCreadie RG, Kelly C, Connolly M, Williams S, Baxter G, Lean M, Paterson JR (2005) Dietary improvement in people with schizophrenia: randomised controlled trial. *Br J Psychiatry* 187:346-51.

McEvoy JP (2005) Prevalence of the metabolic syndrome in patients with schizophre- nia: baseline results from the Clinical Antipsychotic Trials of Intervention Effective- ness (CATIE) schizophrenia trial and comparison with national estimates from NHANES III. *Schizophr. Res.* 80 (1), 19–32.

McGurk SR, Twamley EW, Sitzer DI, McHugo GJ, Mueser KT (2007) A meta-analysis of cognitive remediation in schizophrenia. *Am J Psychiatry* 164:1791–1802.

McGurk SR, Mueser KT, DeRosa TJ, Wolfe R (2009) Work, recovery, and comorbidity in schizophrenia: a randomized controlled trial of cognitive remediation. *Schizophr Bull* 35:319–335.

Mechelli A, Prata DP, Fu CH, et al. (2008) The effects of neuregulin1 on brain function in controls and patients with schizophrenia and bipolar disorder. *Neuroimage* 42: 817–826.

Medalia A, Revheim N, Casey M (2001) The remediation of problem-solving skills in schizophrenia. *Schizophrenia Bulletin* 27, 259–267.

Medalia A, Choi J (2009) Cognitive remediation in schizophrenia. *Neuropsychol* Rev 19:353–364.

Medalia A, Saperstein AM (2013) Does cognitive remediation for schizophrenia improve functional outcomes? *Curr Opin Psychiatry* 26(2):151-7. doi: 10.1097/YCO.0b013e32835dcbd4.

Mego DM, Omori JM, Hanley JF (1988) Transdermal scopolamine as a cause of transient psychosis in two elderly patients. *South Med.* J. 81:394–395.

Mehta MA, Goodyer IM, Sahakian BJ (2004) Methylphenidate improves working memory and set-shifting in AD/HD: relationships to baseline memory capacity. *J Child Psychol Psychiatry* 45: 293-305.

Millan MJ (2000) Improving the treatment of schizophrenia: focus on serotonin (5 HT) (1A) receptors. *J Pharmacol Exp Ther,* 295, pp. 853–861.

Miller EK (1999) The prefrontal cortex: complex neural properties for complex behavior. *Neuron* 22, 15–17.

Miyamoto E (2006) Molecular mechanism of neuronal plasticity: Induction and maintenance of long-term potentiation in the hippocampus. *J. Pharmacol. Sci* 100, pp. 433–442.

Moghaddam B, Adams BW (1998) Reversal of phencyclidine effects by a group II metabotropic glutamate receptor agonist in rats. *Science*, 281, pp. 1349–1352.

Morrison PD, Zois V, McKeown DA, Lee TD, Holt DW, Powell JF, Kapur S, Murray RM (2009) The acute effects of synthetic intravenous Delta9-tetrahydrocannabinol on psychosis, mood and cognitive functioning. *Psychol Med* 39(10):1607-16. doi: 10.1017/S0033291709005522.

Müller U, Rowe JB, Rittman T, Lewis C, Robbins TW, Sahakian BJ (2013) Effects of modafinil on non-verbal cognition, task enjoyment and creative thinking in healthy volunteers. *Neuropharmacology* 64:490-5. doi: 10.1016/j.neuropharm.2012.07.009.

Murthy NV, Mahncke H, Wexler BE, Maruff P, Inamdar A, Zucchetto M, Lund J, Shabbir S, Shergill S, Keshavan M, Kapur S, Laruelle M, Alexander R (2012) Computerized cognitive remediation training for schizophrenia: an open label, multi-site, multinational methodology study. *Schizophr Res* 139(1-3):87-91. doi: 10.1016/j.schres.2012.01.042.

Nagy Z, Westerberg H, Klingberg T (2004) Maturation of white matter is associated with the development of cognitive functions during childhood. *Journal of Cognitive Neuroscience*, 16, pp. 1227–1233.

Need AC, Keefe RS, Ge D, Grossman I, Dickson S, McEvoy JP, Goldstein DB (2009) Pharmacogenetics of antipsychotic response in the CATIE trial: a candidate gene analysis. *Eur J Hum Genet* 17(7):946-57. doi: 10.1038/ejhg.2008.264.

Newcomer JW, Farber NB, Jevtovic-Todorovic V, Selke G, Melson AK, Hershey T, Craft S, Olney JW (1999) Ketamine-induced NMDA receptor hypofunction as a model of memory impairment and psychosis. *Neuropsychopharmacology* 20, pp. 106–118.

Newcomer JW (2005) Second-generation (atypical) antipsychotics and metabolic effects: a comprehensive literature review. *CNS Drugs.*;19 Suppl 1:1-93. Review.

Nolan SF, Roman MW (2012) Lurasidone (latuda®): an atypical antipsychotic. *Issues Ment Health Nurs* 33(5):342-3. doi: 10.3109/01612840.2012.669025. Review.

Nolte S, Wong D, Lachford G (2004) Amphetamines for schizophrenia. *Cochrane Database Syst Rev* (4):CD004964.

Nuechterlein KH, Green MF, Kern RS, Baade LE, Barch DM, Cohen JD, Essock S, Fenton WS, Frese FJ 3rd, Gold JM, Goldberg T, Heaton RK, Keefe RS, Kraemer H, Mesholam-Gately R, Seidman LJ, Stover E, Weinberger DR, Young AS, Zalcman S, Marder SR (2008) The MATRICS Consensus Cognitive Battery, part 1: test selection, reliability, and validity. *Am J Psychiatry* 165(2):203-13. doi: 10.1176/appi.ajp.2007.07010042.

Ochoa EL, Li L, McNamee MG (1990) Desensitization of central cholinergic mechanisms and neuroadaptation to nicotine. *Mol Neurobiol* 4:251–287.

O'Donnell P (2012) Cortical disinhibition in the neonatal ventral hippocampal lesion model of schizophrenia: new vistas on possible therapeutic approaches. *Pharmacol Ther* 133(1):19-25. doi: 10.1016/j.pharmthera.2011.07.005. Review.

Olesen P.J., Nagy Z., Westerberg H., Klingberg T. (2003) Combined analysis of DTI and fMRI data reveals a joint maturation of white and grey matter in a fronto-parietal network. *Cognitive Brain Research,* 18, pp. 48–57.

Olincy A, Harris JG, Johnson LL, Pender V, Kongs S, Allensworth D, Ellis J, Zerbe GO, Leonard S, Stevens KE, Stevens JO, Martin L, Adler LE, Soti F, Kem WR, Freedman R (2006) Proof-of-concept trial of an alpha7 nicotinic agonist in schizophrenia. *Arch Gen Psychiatry* 63(6):630-8.

Olney JW, Newcomer JW, Farber NB (1999) NMDA receptor hypofunction model of schizophrenia. *J. Psychiatr. Res* 33, pp. 523–533.

Oranje B, Glenthøj BY (2012) Clonidine Normalizes Sensorimotor Gating Deficits in Patients With Schizophrenia on Stable Medication. *Schizophr Bull.* Aug 27. [Epub ahead of print] PubMed PMID: 22750632.

Parasuraman R (1998) *The attentive brain*. MIT Press, MA, USA.

Patterson TL, Mausbach BT, McKibbin C, Goldman S, Bucardo J, Jeste DV (2006) Functional adaptation skills training (FAST): a randomized trial of a psychosocial intervention for middle-aged and older patients with chronic psychotic disorders. *Schizophr Res* 86:291–299

Patterson F, Jepson C, Strasser AA, Loughead J, Perkins KA, Gur RC, Frey JM, Siegel S, Lerman C (2009) Varenicline improves mood and cognition during smoking abstinence. *Biol Psychiatry* 65(2): 144-9.

Pedersen CA, Gibson CM, Rau SW, et al (2011) Intranasal oxytocin reduces & psychotic symptoms and improves Theory of Mind and social perception in schizophrenia. *Schizophr Res* 132:50 – 53.

Perl O, Strous RD, Dranikov A, Chen R, Fuchs S (2006) Low levels of alpha7-nicotinic acetylcholine receptor mRNA on peripheral blood lymphocytes in schizophrenia and its association with illness severity. *Neuropsychobiology* 53(2):88-93.

Perry E, Walker M, Grace J, Perry R (1999) Acetylcholine in mind: a neurotransmitter correlate of consciousness? *Trends Neurosci.* 22:273–280.

Pierri JN, Volk CL, Auh S, Sampson A, Lewis DA (2001) Decreased somal size of deep layer 3 pyramidal neurons in the prefrontal cortex of subjects with schizophrenia. *Arch Gen Psychiatry* 58(5):466-73.

Pietrzak RH, Snyder PJ, Maruff P (2010a) Amphetamine-related improvement in executive function in patients with chronic schizophrenia is modulated by practice effects. *Schizophr Res* 124(1-3):176-82. doi: 10.1016/j.schres.2010.09.012.

Pietrzak RH, Snyder PJ, Maruff P (2010b) Use of an acute challenge with d-amphetamine to model cognitive improvement in chronic schizophrenia. *Hum Psychopharmacol* 25(4):353-8. doi: 10.1002/hup.1118.

Pilling S, Bebbington P, Kuipers E, Garety P, Geddes J, Martindale B, Orbach G, Morgan C (2002) Psychological treatments in schizophrenia: II. Meta-analyses of randomized controlled trials of social skills training and cognitive remediation. *Psychol Med* 32(5):783-91.

Pin JP, Acher F (2002) The metabotropic glutamate receptors: Structure, activation mechanism and pharmacology. *Curr. Drug Target CNS Neurol. Disord* 1, pp. 297–317.

Poirier MF, Canceil O, Baylé F, Millet B, Bourdel MC, Moatti C, Olié JP, Attar-Lévy D (2002) Prevalence of smoking in psychiatric patients. *Prog Neuropsychopharmacol Biol Psychiatry* 26(3):529-37.

Porto PR, Oliveira L, Mari J, Volchan E, Figueira I, Ventura P (2009) Does cognitive behavioral therapy change the brain? A systematic review of neuroimaging in anxiety disorders. *J Neuropsychiatry Clin Neurosci* 21:114–125. doi:10.1176/appi.neuropsych.21.2.114

Prilipko O, Huynh N, Schwartz S, Tantrakul V, Kim JH, Peralta AR, Kushida C, Paiva T, Guilleminault C (2011) Task positive and default mode networks during a parametric working memory task in obstructive sleep apnea patients and healthy controls. *Sleep* 34(3):293-301A.

Prilipko O, Huynh N, Schwartz S, Tantrakul V, Kushida C, Paiva T, Guilleminault C (2012) The effects of CPAP treatment on task positive and default mode networks in obstructive sleep apnea patients: an fMRI study. *PLoS One* 7(12):e47433. doi: 10.1371/journal.pone.0047433.

Randrup A, Munkvad (1967) Stereotyped activities produced by amphetamine in several animal species and man. *Psychopharmacologia* 11:300-310.

Rapoport JL, Buchsbaum MS, Weingartner H, Zahn TP, Ludlow C, Mikkelsen EJ (1980) Dextroamphetamine: Its cognitive and behavioral effects in normal and hyperactive boys and normal men. *Arch Gen Psychiatry* 37:933-943.

Raznahan A, Lee Y, Long R, Greenstein D, Clasen L, Addington A, Rapoport JL, Giedd JN (2011) Common functional polymorphisms of DISC1 and cortical maturation in typically developing children and adolescents. *Mol Psychiatry* 16(9):917-26. doi: 10.1038/mp.2010.72.

Rees TM, Brimijoin S (2003) The role of acetylcholinesterase in the pathogenesis of Alzheimer's disease. *Drugs Today* (Barc) 39:75-83.

Ressler KJ, Rothbaum BO, Tannenbaum L, Anderson P, Graap K, Zimand E, Hodges L, Davis M (2004) Cognitive enhancers as adjuncts to psychotherapy: use of D-cycloserine in phobic individuals to facilitate extinction of fear. *Arch Gen Psychiatry* 61:1136-1144.

Ribeiz SR, Bassitt DP, Arrais JA (2010) Cholinesterase inhibitors as adjunctive therapy in patients with schizophrenia and schizoaffective disorder: a review and meta-analysis of the literature. *CNS Drugs* 24:303-17.

Risbood V, Lee JR, Roche-Desilets J, Fuller MA (2012) Lurasidone: an atypical antipsychotic for schizophrenia. *Ann Pharmacother* 46(7-8):1033-46. doi: 10.1345/aph.1M721. Review.

Roche Laboratories N (1998) *Tasmar (tolcapone) package insert.* Nutley, NJ.

Rosenfeld AJ, Lieberman JA, Jarskog LF (2011) Oxytocin, dopamine, and the amygdala: a neurofunctional model of social cognitive deficits in schizophrenia. *Schizophr Bull* 37(5):1077-87. doi: 10.1093/schbul/sbq015.

Rosenthal MH, Bryant SL (2004) Benefits of adjunct modafinil in an open-label, pilot study in patients with schizophrenia. *Clin Neuropharmacol* 27(1):38-43.

Rusted JM, Trawley S (2006) Comparable effects of nicotine in smokers and nonsmokers on a prospective memory task. *Neuropsychopharmacology* 31(7): 1545-9.

Sacco KA, Termine A, Seyal A, Dudas MM, Vessicchio JC, Krishnan-Sarin S, Jatlow PI, Wexler BE, George TP (2005) Effects of cigarette smoking on spatial working memory and attentional deficits in schizophrenia: involvement of nicotinic receptor mechanisms. *Arch Gen Psychiatry* 62(6): 649-59.

Sacks FM (2004) Metabolic syndrome: epidemiology and consequences. *J Clin Psychiatry* 65 Suppl 18:3-12. Review.

Santos NC, Costa P, Ruano D, Macedo A, Soares MJ, Valente J, Pereira AT, Azevedo MH, Palha JA (2012) Revisiting thyroid hormones in schizophrenia. *J Thyroid Res.*;2012:569147. doi: 10.1155/2012/569147.

Sapara A, Cooke M, Fannon D, Francis A, Buchanan RW, Anilkumar AP, Barkataki I, Aasen I, Kuipers E, Kumari V (2007) Prefrontal cortex and insight in schizophrenia: a volumetric MRI study. *Schizophr Res* 89(1-3):22-34.

Sarter M, Nelson CL, Bruno JP (2005) Cortical cholinergic transmission and cortical information processing in schizophrenia. *Schizophr. Bull.* 31:117–138.

Sartory G, Zorn C, Groetzinger G, Windgassen K (2005) Computerized cognitive remediation improves verbal learning and processing speed in schizophrenia. *Schizophrenia Research* 75, 219–223.

Sawaguchi T, Matsumura M, Kubota K (1990a) Effects of dopamine antagonists on neuronal activity related to a delated response task in monkey prefrontal cortex. *J Neurophysiol* 63(6): 1401-12.

Sawaguchi T, Matsumura M, Kubota K (1990b) Catecholaminergic effects on neuronal activity related to a delayed response task in monkey prefrontal cortex. *J Neurophysiol* 63(6): 1385-99.

Saxena S, Gorbis E, O'Neill J, Baker SK, Mandelkern MA, Maidment KM, Chang S, Salamon N, Brody AL, Schwartz JM, London ED (2009) Rapid effects of brief intensive cognitive-behavioral therapy on brain glucose metabolism in obsessive-compulsive disorder. *Mol Psychiatry* 14:197–205. doi:10.1038/sj.mp.4002134

Scahill L, Chappell PB, Kim YS, Schultz RT, Katsovich L, Shepherd E, Arnsten AFT, Cohen DJ, Leckman JF (2001) Guanfacine in the treatment of children with tic disorders and ADHD: a placebo-controlled study. *Am J Psychiatry* 158:1067–1074.

Schoepp DD, Marek GJ (2002) Preclinical pharmacology of mglu2/3 receptor agonists: Novel agents for schizophrenia? *Curr. Drug Target CNS Neurol. Disord* 1, pp. 215–225.

Scoriels L, Barnett JH, Soma PK, Sahakian BJ, Jones PB (2012) Effects of modafinil on cognitive functions in first episode psychosis. *Psychopharmacology* (Berl) 220(2):249-58. doi: 10.1007/s00213-011-2472-4.

Seeman MV (2011) Antipsychotic-induced amenorrhea. *J Ment Health* 20(5):484-91. doi: 10.3109/09638237.2011.586741. Review.

Segev A, Lev-Ran S (2012) Neurocognitive functioning and cannabis use in schizophrenia. *Curr Pharm Des* 18(32):4999-5007.

Sekine Y, Takei N, Suzuki K, Nakamura K, Tsuchiya KJ, Takebayashi K, Toulopoulou T, Mori N (2005) Effective adjunctive use of pergolide with quetiapine for cognitive impairment and negative symptoms in schizophrenia. *J Clin Psychopharmacol* 25(3):281-3. PubMed PMID: 15876913.

Shirey JK, Brady AE, Jones PJ et al (2009) A selective allosteric potentiator of the M1 muscarinic acetylcholine receptor increases activity of medial prefrontal cortical neurons and restores impairments in reversal learning. *J Neurosci* 29:14271–14286.

Siegel BV Jr, Trestman RL, O'Flaithbheartaigh S, Mitropoulou V, Amin F, Kirrane R, Silverman J, Schmeidler J, Keefe RS, Siever LJ (1996) D-amphetamine challenge effects on Wisconsin Card Sort Test. Performance in schizotypal personality disorder. *Schizophr Res* 20(1-2):29-32.

Simonelli-Muñoz AJ, Fortea MI, Salorio P, Gallego-Gomez JI, Sánchez-Bautista S, Balanza S (2012) Dietary habits of patients with schizophrenia: a self-reported questionnaire survey. *Int J Ment Health Nurs* 21(3):220-8. doi: 10.1111/j.1447-0349.2012.00821.x.

Singh J, Kour K, Jayaram MB (2012) Acetylcholinesterase inhibitors for schizophrenia.*Cochrane Database Syst Rev* 1:CD007967.

Sitzer DI, Twamley EW, Patterson TL, Jeste DV (2008) Multivariate predictors of social skills performance in middle-aged and older out-patients with schizophrenia spectrum disorders. *Psychol Med* 38(5):755-63.

Smith RC, Lindenmayer JP, Davis JM, Cornwell J, Noth K, Gupta S, Sershen H, Lajtha A (2009) Cognitive and antismoking effects of varenicline in patients with schizophrenia or schizoaffective disorder. *Schizophr Res* 110(1-3): 149-55.

Snyder SH (1973) Amphetamine psychosis: a "model" schizophrenia mediated by catecholamines. *Am J Psychiatry* 130:61-67.

Stiles J, Jernigan TL (2010) The basics of brain development. *Neuropsychology* Review 20, pp. 327–348.

Subramaniam K, Luks TL, Fisher M, Simpson GV, Nagarajan S, Vinogradov S (2012) Computerized cognitive training restores neural activity within the reality monitoring network in schizophrenia. *Neuron* 73(4):842-53. doi: 10.1016/j.neuron.2011.12.024.

Sumiyoshi T, Matsui M, Yamashita I, Nohara S, Uehara T, Kurachi M, Meltzer HY (2000) Effect of adjunctive treatment with serotonin-1A agonist tandospirone on memory functions in schizophrenia. *J Clin Psychopharmacol* 20(3):386-8.

Sumiyoshi T, Matsui M, Yamashita I, Nohara S, Kurachi M, Uehara T, Sumiyoshi S, Sumiyoshi C, Meltzer HY (2001a) The effect of tandospirone, a serotonin(1A) agonist, on memory function in schizophrenia. *Biol Psychiatry* 49(10):861-8.

Sumiyoshi T, Matsui M, Nohara S, Yamashita I, Kurachi M, Sumiyoshi C, Jayathilake K, Meltzer HY (2001b) Enhancement of cognitive performance in schizophrenia by addition of tandospirone to neuroleptic treatment. *Am J Psychiatry* 158(10):1722-5

Sumiyoshi T, Park S, Jayathilake K, Roy A, Ertugrul A, Meltzer HY (2007) Effect of buspirone, a serotonin1A partial agonist, on cognitive function in schizophrenia: a randomized, double-blind, placebo-controlled study. *Schizophr Res* 95(1-3):158-68.

Swanson LW (1982) The projections of the ventral tegmental area and adjacent regions: a combined fluorescent retrograde tracer and immunofluorescence study in the rat. *Brain Res Bull* 9(1-6):321-53.

Swerdlow NR, Hartman PL, Auerbach PP (1997) Changes in sensorimotor inhibition across the menstrual cycle: implications for neuropsychiatric disorders. *Biol Psychiatry* 41(4):452-60.

Swerdlow NR (2011) Are we studying and treating schizophrenia correctly? *Schizophr Res* 130(1-3):1-10. doi: 10.1016/j.schres.2011.05.004.

Swerdlow NR (2012) Beyond antipsychotics: pharmacologically-augmented cognitive therapies (PACTs) for schizophrenia. *Neuropsychopharmacology* 37(1):310-1. doi: 10.1038/npp.2011.195.

Takahashi KI, Shimizu T, Sugita T, Saito Y, Takahashi Y, Hishikawa Y (1998) Prevalence of sleep-related respiratory disorders in 101 schizophrenic inpatients. *Psychiatry Clin Neurosci* 52(2):229-31.

Takayanagi Y, Cascella NG, Sawa A, Eaton WW (2012) Diabetes is associated with lower global cognitive function in schizophrenia. *Schizophr Res* 142(1-3):183-7. doi: 10.1016/j.schres.2012.08.034.

Tamminga CA, Holcomb HH, Gao X, Lahti AC (1995) Glutamate pharmacology and the treatment of schizophrenia: Current status and future directions. *Int. Clin. Psychopharmacol* 10 (Suppl. 3), pp. 29–37.

Tan HY, Callicott JH, Weinberger DR (2009) Prefrontal cognitive systems in schizophrenia: towards human genetic brain mechanisms. *Cogn Neuropsychiatry* 14(4-5):277-98. doi: 10.1080/13546800903091665.

Tan HY, Chen AG, Kolachana B, Apud JA, Mattay VS, Callicott JH, Chen Q, Weinberger DR (2012) Effective connectivity of AKT1-mediated dopaminergic working memory networks and pharmacogenetics of antidopaminergic treatment. *Brain* 135(Pt 5):1436-45. doi: 10.1093/brain/aws068.

Taylor FB, Russo J (2001) Comparing guanfacine and dextroamphetamine for the treatment of adult attention deficit-hyperactivity disorder. *J Clin Psychopharmacol* 21:223–228.

Teng CT, Demetrio FN (2006) Memantine may acutely improve cognition and have a mood stabilizing effect in treatment-resistant bipolar disorder. *Rev Bras Psiquiatr* 28(3):252-4.

Torres IJ, Keedy S, Marlow-O'Connor M, Beenken B, Goldman MB (2009) Neuropsychological impairment in patients with schizophrenia and evidence of hyponatremia and polydipsia. *Neuropsychology* 23(3):307-14. doi: 10.1037/a0014481.

Tsai GE, Yang P, Chung LC, Lange N, Coyle JT (1998) D-serine added to antipsychotics for the treatment of schizophrenia. *Biol. Psychiatry* 44, pp. 1081–1089.

Tsai GE, Yang P, Chung LC, Tsai IC, Tsai CW, Coyle JT (1999) D-serine added to clozapine for the treatment of schizophrenia. *Am. J. Psychiatry* 156, pp. 1822–1825.

Tsai GE, Yang P, Chang YC, Chong MY (2005) D-alanine added to antipsychotics for the treatment of schizophrenia. *Biol. Psychiatry* 59 (3), pp. 230–234.

Tufts Center for the Study of Drug Development, 2006: Cost to Develop New Biotech Products is Estimated to Average $1.2 billion. *Tufts CSDD Impact Report 8.*

Twamley EW, Savla GN, Zurhellen CH, Heaton RK, Jeste DV (2008) Development and Pilot Testing of a Novel Compensatory Cognitive Training Intervention for People with Psychosis. *Am J Psychiatr Rehabil.* 11(2):144-163.

Twamley EW (2010) Compensatory cognitive training for patients with psychosis. *Schizophr Res;* 117:142–143.

Twamley EW, Burton CZ, Vella L (2011) Compensatory cognitive training for psychosis: who benefits? Who stays in treatment? *Schizophr Bull* 37 Suppl 2:S55-62. doi: 10.1093/schbul/sbr059.

Twamley EW, Vella L, Burton CZ, Heaton RK, Jeste DV (2012) Compensatory cognitive training for psychosis: effects in a randomized controlled trial. *J Clin Psychiatry* 73(9):1212-9. doi: 10.4088/JCP.12m07686. Epub 2012 Aug 7. PubMed PMID: 22939029.

Ueland T, Rund BR (2004) A controlled randomized treatment study: the effects of a cognitive remediation program on adolescents with early onset psychosis. *Acta Psychiatr. Scand* 109(1):70–74.

Vaillancourt C, Cyr M, Rochford J, Boksa P, Di Paolo T (2002) Effects of ovariectomy and estradiol on acoustic startle responses in rats. *Pharmacol Biochem Behav* 74(1):103-9.

Van Citters AD, Pratt SI, Jue K, Williams G, Miller PT, Xie H, Bartels SJ (2010) A pilot evaluation of the In SHAPE individualized health promotion intervention for adults with mental illness. *Community Ment Health J* 46(6):540-52. doi: 10.1007/s10597-009-9272-x.

Van den Buuse M, Eikelis N (2001) Estrogen increases prepulse inhibition of acoustic startle in rats. *Eur J Pharmacol* 425(1):33-41.

van der Kemp WJ, Klomp DW, Kahn RS, Luijten PR, Hulshoff Pol HE (2012) A meta-analysis of the polyunsaturated fatty acid composition of erythrocyte membranes in schizophrenia. *Schizophr Res* 141(2-3):153-61. doi: 10.1016/j.schres.2012.08.014.

van Os J, Bak M, Hanssen M, et al (2002) Cannabis use and psychosis: a longitudinal population-based study. *American Journal of Epidemiology,* 156, 319– 327.

van Rossum J (1966) The significance of dopamine-receptor blockade for the mechanism of action of neuroleptic drugs. *Arch Int Pharmacodyn Ther* 160:492-494.

Velligan DI, Draper M, Stutes D, Maples N, Mintz J, Tai S, et al. (2009) Multimodal cognitive therapy: Combining treatments that bypass cognitive deficits and deal with reasoning and appraisal biases. *Schizophrenia Bulletin, 35*, 884–893.

Vinogradov S (2012a) Neuroscience-informed cognitive training in recent onset schizophrenia using laptop computer. *8th Int. Conf. Early Psychosis*, San Francisco, CA.

Vinogradov S, Fisher M, de Villers-Sidani E. (2012b) Cognitive training for impaired neural systems in neuropsychiatric illness. *Neuropsychopharmacology* 37:43–76.

Volpicelli LA, Levey AI (2004) Muscarinic acetylcholine receptor subtypes in cerebral cortex and hippocampus. *Prog. Brain Res.* 145:59–66.

Waldstein SR, Katzel LI (2006) Interactive relations of central versus total obesity and blood pressure to cognitive function. *Int J Obes* (Lond). Jan;30(1):201-7. PubMed PMID: 16231030.

Wang LJ, Ree SC, Huang YS, Hsiao CC, Chen CK (2013) Adjunctive effects of aripiprazole on metabolic profiles: comparison of patients treated with olanzapine to patients treated with other atypical antipsychotic drugs. *Prog Neuropsychopharmacol Biol Psychiatry* 40:260-6. doi: 10.1016/j.pnpbp.2012.10.010.

Wang Y, Fang Y, Shen Y, Xu Q (2010). Analysis of association between the catechol-O-methyltransferase (COMT) gene and negative symptoms in chronic schizophrenia. *Psychiatry Res.* 30;179(2):147-50.

Weiser M, Heresco-Levy U, Davidson M, Javitt DC, Werbeloff N, Gershon AA, Abramovich Y, Amital D, Doron A, Konas S, Levkovitz Y, Liba D, Teitelbaum A, Mashiach M, Zimmerman Y (2012) A multicenter, add-on randomized controlled trial of low-dose d-serine for negative and cognitive symptoms of schizophrenia. *J Clin Psychiatry* 73(6):e728-34. doi: 10.4088/JCP.11m07031.

Weinberger DR, Berman KF, Zee RF (1986) Physiologic dysfunction of dorsolateral prefrontal cortex in schizophrenia. I. Regional cerebral blood flow evidence. *Archives General Psychiatry* 43:114–124.

Williams NM, O'Donovan MC and Owen MJ (2005) Is the dysbindin gene (DTNBP1) a susceptibility gene for schizophrenia? *Schizophr Bull* 31: 800–805.

Wilson PW, Grundy SM (2003a) The metabolic syndrome: a practical guide to origins and treatment: Part II. *Circulation* 108(13):1537-40. Review.

Wilson PW, Grundy SM (2003b) The metabolic syndrome: practical guide to origins and treatment: Part I. *Circulation* 108(12):1422-4. Review.

Winkelman JW (2001) Schizophrenia, obesity, and obstructive sleep apnea. *J Clin Psychiatry* 62(1):8-11.

Wirshing DA, Pierre JM, Wirshing WC (2002) Sleep apnea associated with antipsychotic-induced obesity. *J Clin Psychiatry*. 63(4):369-70.

Wirshing DA (2004) Schizophrenia and obesity: impact of antipsychotic medications. *J Clin Psychiatry* 65 Suppl 18:13-26.

Wise SP, Murray EA, Gerfen CR (1996) The frontal-basal ganglia system in primates. *Crit. Rev. Neurobiol.* 10, 317–356.

Wonodi I, Cassady SL, Adami H, Avila M, Thaker GK (2006) Effects of repeated amphetamine administration on antisaccade in schizophrenia spectrum personality. *Psychiatry Res* 141(3):237-45.

Wulff K, Joyce E (2011) Circadian rhythms and cognition in schizophrenia. *Br J Psychiatry* 198(4):250-2. doi: 10.1192/bjp.bp.110.085068.

Wykes T, van der Gaag M (2001) Is it time to develop a new cognitive therapy for psychosis--cognitive remediation therapy (CRT)? *Clin Psychol Rev.* 21(8):1227-56. Review.

Wykes T, Newton E, Landau S, Rice C, Thompson N, Frangou S (2007) Cognitive remediation therapy (CRT) for young early onset patients with schizophrenia: an exploratory randomized controlled trial. *Schizophr. Res* 94(1–3):221–30.

Wykes T, Huddy V, Cellard C, McGurk SR, Czobor P (2011) A meta-analysis of cognitive remediation for schizophrenia: methodology and effect sizes. *Am J Psychiatry 168*:472–485. doi:10.1176/appi.ajp.2010.10060855

Xiang YT, Weng YZ, Leung CM, Tang WK, Sandor UG (2007) Exploring the clinical and social determinants of prescribing anticholinergic medication for Chinese patients with schizophrenia. *Hum Psychopharmacol* 22(3):173-80.

Zammit, S., Allebeck, P., Andreasson, S., et al (2002) Self reported cannabis use as a risk factor for schizophrenia in Swedish conscripts of 1969: historical cohort study. *BMJ*, 325, 1199– 1201.

Zimmermann U, Kraus T, Himmerich H, Schuld A, Pollmächer T (2003) Epidemiology, implications and mechanisms underlying drug-induced weight gain in psychiatric patients. *J Psychiatr Res* 37(3):193-220. Review.

In: Prefrontal Cortex
Editors: R. O. Collins and J. L. Adams
ISBN 978-1-62618-663-7

Chapter 4

COGNITIVE FUNCTIONING AND PREFRONTAL CORTEX DAMAGE IN CHILDREN AND ADOLESCENTS: CONSEQUENCES, REHABILITATION AND NEURAL PLASTICITY

Ana Luiza Vidal Milioni,[1,2] Priscila Aparecida Rodrigues[1] and Paulo Jannuzzi Cunha[2,3,4]

[1]Institute of Physical Medicine and Rehabilitation (IMREA), Clinics Hospital, School of Medicine, University of São Paulo, Brazil

[2]Laboratory of Psychiatric Neuroimaging (LIM-21)/ Center for Interdisciplinary Research on Applied Neurosciences (NAPNA), School of Medicine, University of São Paulo, Brazil

[3]Interdisciplinary Group on Studies of Alcohol and Drugs (GREA), Institute of Psychiatry, University of São Paulo, Brazil

[4]Equilibrium Program, Institute of Psychiatry, University of São Paulo, Brazil

ABSTRACT

Traumatic brain injury (TBI) is a major problem of public health around the world since it is the first cause of death among children and adolescents in most of the developed countries. TBI is a neurological disorder that results in temporary or permanent changes in motor, cognitive and behavioral areas. TBI is one of the most common kinds of brain injuries in childhood/adolescence, a period in which the prefrontal cortex is in a developing process. The aim of this chapter is to review neuropsychological consequences of TBI in prefrontal cortex during childhood/adolescence, as well as the valid strategies to be adopted that might contribute to a shorter recovery time of the young people in development. The TBI in the prefrontal cortex does not involve motor or sensorial deficits. However, it can cause functional, social and academic impairments. More than a half of these children/adolescents develop a psychiatric disorder with disinhibiting symptoms and inappropriate behavior. Motivational, emotional, attention, perceptive and cognitive functions are mediated by the connections between the prefrontal cortex and the motor areas, the limbic system, the reticular system and the posterior association cortex. Generally, patients with TBI will present cognitive deficits associated with executive functions, decision making, problem solving skills, judgment and impulse control. The consequences of brain injury in childhood/adolescence depend on a variety of factors, such as: the type of brain injury, intensity of the damage, extension, localization, environmental factors, age in which the TBI occurs, premorbid intelligence/cognitive reserve, and stage of cognitive development. For example, dorsolateral lesions have been associated with perseverative behavior, lack of initiative, deficit in ability to sustain and shift attention between stimuli or concepts, problem solving and working memory ("cold" executive functions). It is commonly confused with unmotivated behavior. On the other hand, ventromedial injuries have been associated with conducts based on emotional and social variables, such as inability to respond appropriately to social cues, failure to obey conventional social rules, inhibitory deficits, impulsivity and impaired decision making ("hot" executive functions).

Right after the brain injury, new mechanisms of repair and reorganization of the Central Nervous System (CNS) emerge for an indefinite time period, aiming to reduce and compensate the functional impairment associated with the problem. A new neuronal circuit in the neighbor areas of the brain is established to recover lost functions and consequently to help the accomplishment of activities. The process of restructuring the brain and strengthening the cognitive functions is called neural plasticity and it can improve the prognostic of the subject at any stage of development or adult life.

In most children/adolescents, when the brain injury in the prefrontal cortex happens, special educational needs or changes in the educational environment are necessary. In the meantime, there are promising treatments with stimulant drugs, neuropsychological rehabilitation, and cognitive behavioral therapy strategies. Further studies on neuropsychological rehabilitation are required to define to what extent individuals affected by TBI may have a restoration of premorbid cognitive abilities by making use of these integrated techniques.

Keywords: Prefrontal cortex, brain injury and neurodevelopment

INTRODUCTION

Traumatic brain injury (TBI) is a major problem of public health around the world since it is the first cause of death among children and adolescents in most of the developed countries (Arciniegas, Anderson, Topkoff and McAllister, 2005). In the United States, an estimated 1.4 million people sustain a TBI annually (Dikmen, et al., 2009).

Official Reports suggest that 170 in 100.000 children will suffer a TBI in the US each year (Anderson, Godfrey, Rosenfeld and Catroppa, 2012). It results in temporary or permanent changes in motor, cognitive and behavioral areas. TBI is one of the most common kinds of brain injuries in childhood/adolescence, a period in which the prefrontal cortex is in a developing process.

The two main causes of TBI during childhood/adolescence are traffic accidents and falls. The majority of TBI in children/adolescents are mild, typically with few long-term consequences, however, a significant number of these people will suffer more serious damages and will experience physical, cognitive, educational, functional, emotional and social impairments (Stacin et al., 2002).

The brain areas work together and each part is responsible for one or more specific functions that contribute to more complex cognitive processes. For this reason, an injury in a single area of the brain may affect many functions. Considering this network of complex connections, it is hard to establish a rigid association between a specific region of the brain and a single cognitive function.

Also, especially with children/adolescents, who are still acquiring new skills and brain maturity, the consequences of such damage are much more complex.

The aim of this chapter is to review the neuropsychological consequences of TBI in prefrontal cortex during childhood/adolescence, as well as the valid strategies to be adopted that might contribute to a shorter recovery time of the young people in development.

TBI

Definition and Classification

TBI is a nondegenerative and noncongenital neurological disorder that occurs after an insult to the brain caused by an external mechanical force (Ewing-Cobbs and Bloom, 1999; Koehler, Wilhelm and Shoulson, 2011).

TBI is classified as mild, moderate and severe based upon the alteration of consciousness that follows the injury. The most commonly used scale to measure the level of severity of TBI is the Glasgow Coma Scale. It has a configuration for adults and older children (Table 1) and a different one for nonverbal children, the Pediatric Glasgow Coma Scale for Nonverbal Children (Table 2).

Both scales follow the same score classification: severe TBI is defined as a Glasgow Coma Scale score between 3 and 8, moderate TBI is between 9 and 12 and mild TBI is between 13 and 15.

Table 1. Glasgow Coma Scale

Behavior	Response	Score
Eye opening response	Spontaneously	4
	To speech	3
	To pain	2
	No response	1
Best verbal response	Oriented to time, place and person	5
	Confused	4
	Inappropriate words	3
	Imcomprehensible sounds	2
	No response	1
Best motor response	Obeys commands	6
	Moves to localized pain	5
	Flexion withdrawal from pain	4
	Abnormal flexoin (decorticate)	3
	Abnormal extension (decerebrate)	2
	No response	1
Total score	Best response	15
	Comatose client	8 or less
	Totally unresponsive	3

Table 2. Pediatric Glasgow Coma Scale For Nonverbal Children

Behavior	Response	Score
Eye opening	Spontaneous	4
	To speech	3
	To pain	2
	No response	1
Verbal Response	Coos, babbles	5
	Irritable cry	4
	Crien to pain	3
	Moans to pain	2
	No response	1
Motor Response	Follows commands	6
	Localizes pain	5
	Withdraws to pain	4
	Decorticate flexion	3
	Decerebrate extension	2
	No response	1

There are two main types of TBI: open or closed. The Open-Type TBI occurs when an object penetrates the skull or when the skull is broken, like in wounds caused by fire guns or falls with bone perforation (Ewing-Cobbs and Bloom, 1999). In addition to physically damaging the brain, open head injuries are more likely to get an infection, which may complicate the condition. The closed-type TBI occurs when the brain collides with the inside of the skull after a crash. Even though sometimes there are no visible signals of injury, the brain can swell inside the skull pressuring delicate neighbor tissues. In this case, there are no damages to the bone structure. It generally occurs after falls, car accidents, electric shocks and others (Dikmen et al., 2009).

Both types of TBI frequently produce prefrontal lesions and disconnect this area from associated cortical and subcortical areas.

Neurodevelopment

The maturation of a child´s brain is a complex process, in which the brain grows and produces several behavioral changes, in order to adapt to the surrounding world (Aamodt and Wang, 2011). The brain of a newborn baby has higher synaptic density than the adult brain (García-Molina, Ensenat-

Cantallops, Tirapu-Ustarroz and Roig-Rovira, 2009). After birth, however, the synapses form rapidly in all areas of the brain (Johnson, 2001). At the age of 3, the synaptic density reaches its peak at levels 50% higher than those found in adults (Bruer, 1998). However, it is important to remember that the peak density of synapses occur at different ages in different areas (Johnson, 2001). In this period, synaptic production outpaces the synaptic elimination and the majority of synapses are formed. This process of synaptogenesis is followed by a posterior period of synaptic pruning, in which both the environment and personal experiences play important roles (Blackmore, 2011).

Executive Functions

Luria (1973) proposes that the cognitive functions and the mental processes are organized in systems that embrace specific brain areas. Each of these areas (in a constant interaction with the others) plays a role in the functional system. According to the author's theory, there are 3 functional units in the brain. The first one is the arousal-motivation unit and refers to the limbic and reticular systems. The second unit is related with receiving, processing and storing information and encompasses the temporal, parietal and occipital lobes. Finally, the third unit is in charge of programming, controlling and verifying mental activity and is located in the frontal lobe (Chan, Shum, Toulopoulou and Chen, 2008). Within the frontal lobe, the prefrontal cortex is considered by Luria as the regulator of mental activity and behavior, a structure that organizes intellectual activity, programs the act and the checks its performance (Luria, 1973). By this perception, the author conceptualized what is presently referred as executive functions.

Executive functions are high-level cognitive abilities that control and regulate other abilities and behaviors. They can be divided in two categories: "hot" and "cold" executive functions. The "hot" executive functions involve emotionally and motivationally influenced decisions and includes the abilities of self-regulation, emotional control and theory of mind. The ventromedial and the orbitofrontal areas are responsible for the "hot" executive functions. The "cold" executive functions, on the other hand, are localized in the dorsolateral and frontostriatal areas and consist of purely cognitive abilities, such as problem solving, mental flexibility, inhibitory control, attention and working memory (Fonseca et al., 2012).

The development of cognitive functions along the childhood and adolescence makes the subject able to process information, regulate actions and make behavior adjustments according to feedbacks from the environment.

According to recent studies, the development of the executive functions begins early in life. At the age of 8 months the baby already reminds simple representations (Reznick, Morrow, Goldman and Snyder, 2004). At this age, when the baby is playing with a toy and someone hides it, he will seek for the object. During the first year of life the skill of inhibition, another kind of executive function, emerges (García-Molina et al., 2009). It can be exemplified by the fact that children at this age have the ability to interrupt a pleasure activity to attend the demand of an adult.

The development of the executive functions is nearly connected to the maturation of the prefrontal cortex (García-Molina et al., 2009; Reznick, Morrow, Goldman and Snyder, 2004; Gogtay et al., 2004). The prefrontal grey matter has its volume increased until the age of 11 in boys and 12 in girls (Blakemore, 2010). The age difference between genders may be explained by an interaction involving puberty hormones and the grey matter development. After that, the grey matter density starts to decrease (Figure 1), reflecting the neural pruning process, a neurological regulatory process by which certain neurons and synapses are removed, leaving only efficient synaptic configuration. Imaging studies found regional nonlinear changes in grey matter during childhood and adolescence (Gogtay et al., 2004). On the other hand, the prefrontal white matter remains on developing process during the entire childhood and adolescence, ceasing only in the second decade of life. The growth is associated to the myelination in the cortico-subcortical pathways that are associated with this brain area. It is higher in the prefrontal dorsolateral area and smaller in the prefrontal orbitofrontal regions (García-Molina et al., 2009).

Prefrontal Cortex

Prefrontal cortex seems to play a major role in the multisynaptic integration of emotion, action and experience. All the prefrontal cortex participates in this process, but the paralimbic components have closer connection with emotion and aspects of visceral functions. The lateral part of orbitofrontal cortex (Figure 2 FOC) seems to be more closely related to sensitivity to punishment whereas it medial part seems more closely related to reward (Schore, 2009).

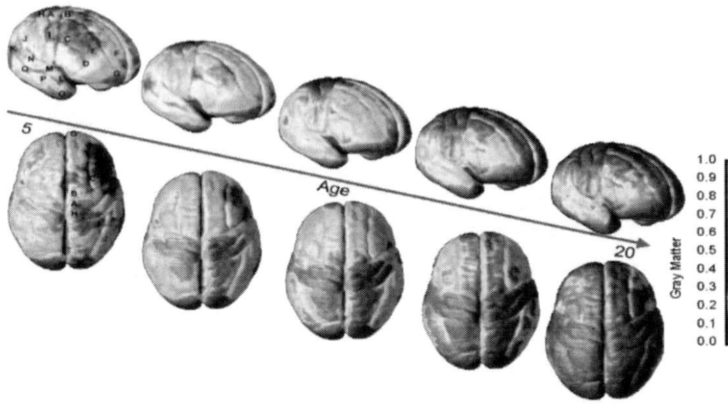

Figure 1. Right lateral and top views of the density decrease on the grey matter´s volume over the cortical surface along the maturation process (Gogtay et al., 2004).

The dorsolateral prefrontal cortex (Figure 2 F1 + F2), together with other connected areas, is especially involved with the traditional executive functions: working memory, planning ability and problem solving (Johnson, 2001). Finally, the ventral prefrontal cortex (Figure 2 FMC + F3t + F3o) is connected with brain regions related to emotional processing and it is responsible for behavior regulation (Johnson, 2001).

TBI AND NEURODEVELOPMENT

The sequelae of TBI during childhood/adolescence may include impairments in language, motor skills, processing speed, attention, learning, memory, social functions and behavioral control. These deficits may restrict the subject's ability to manage activities of daily life appropriate to life stage, for example, education and employment in the future (Anderson, Brown and Newitt, 2010; Fay et al., 1994).

In the past it was argued that the prognosis after TBI was better in the immature brain because of the neural plasticity. This idea was initially proposed by Margaret Kenard in 1936, when studying primates (Cicchetti and Curtis, 2006).

It was found that motor impairments after unilateral motor cortex injury had better prognosis in infant than in adult monkeys. This theory was generalized to humans in claiming that children would sustain less impairment and would recover better after brain injury than adults (Dennis, 2010). The theory was named "Kenard Principle". However, in 1980 decade, studies pointed that despite the fact that the former concept is right, there are more factors to consider before taking a conclusion (Anderson et al., 1997; Kolb, Gibb and Gorny, 2000).

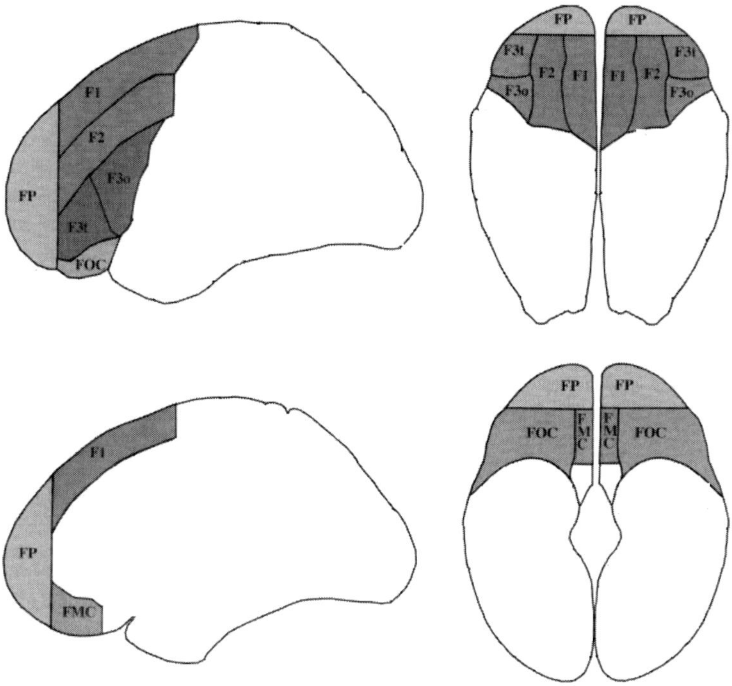

Figure 2. Parcellation units comprising the prefrontal cortical (PFC) regions of interest: frontal pole (FP; orange), dorsolateral PFC (F1 + F2; green), ventrolateral PFC (F3t + F3o; pink), ventromedial PFC (FMC; blue), orbital PFC (FOC; grey).

From a cognitive perspective, the younger the age at injury, the less consolidated are the abilities of the subject. Some of the cognitive skills are not yet established and future acquisition may be compromised.

When it occurs, usually the damage is not very observable in the beginning of the recovery process and the impairments emerge with time, when the children/adolescents starts showing poor or delayed skills acquisition and discrepancies between people of their age (Forsyth and Kirkham, 2012). For example, preadolescents with TBI usually have less improvement in writing than other adolescents who had TBI at an older age since the second group had already established the ability whereas the first one was still acquiring it. Studies point that recovery in motor and visual-spatial functions is slower in younger adolescents than in older ones for the same reason (Thompson et al., 1994). Acquiring developmental abilities over the injury is always a challenge to the brain, which has to adapt its functioning in diverse forms (Anderson et al., 1997).

Once that the prefrontal cortex area is one of the last to become mature during the neurodevelopment, children/adolescents who had a brain injury in this region do not have all functions connected to this area yet established. For this reason, the maturation of the executive functions, the prime function of the prefrontal cortex, may have unexpected outcomes.

TBI in Prefrontal Cortex

Prefrontal cortex damage usually has little overt effects: the person can still walk, perceive and the cognitive impairments are not always evident in short conversations. However, it causes much cognitive impairments, such as: deficit in attention, memory (Voytek and Knight, 2010; Tsuchida and Fellows, 2009) and decision making processes, excessive behavioral rigidity and perseveration, lack of empathy and inhibitory control, inappropriate social behavior (Lovell and Franzen, 1994). Interpersonal skills, judgment, socially appropriated behavior and moral conduct are related to the ability to transcend an egocentric point of view and to regulate behaviors according to the feelings and reactions of others. The impairments on this ability are particularly pronounced if prefrontal damage is acquired early in life or centered in orbitofrontal cortex (Figure 2 FOC).

Brain injury in orbitofrontal area (Figure 2 FOC) also presents lack of self-control, emotional outbursts and generalized disinhibition, deficits in selective attention and problem solving (Schore, 2009).

Patients with damage in the ventromedial (Figure 2 FMC) components of prefrontal cortex usually prefer short-term gains in tasks in which the best strategy would be based on delayed gratifications. The absence of planning and impaired decision-making in these patients is associated with a perseverative impulse to seek immediate gratification.

Dorsolateral damage (Figure 2 F1 + F2), is related to impaired ability to shift conceptual sets, excessive behavioral rigidity and perseveration.

Prefrontal cortex damage is associated with the term “dysexecutive syndrome” because it is characterized by impairments in several cognitive subdomains involving executive functions, as explained before. However, dysexecutive syndrome may be more characterized by specific alterations, depending on the specific brain region affected.

Anderson, Jacobs and Anderson (2010) suggest a list of tests that evaluate the executive functions in children/adolescents. Attentional Control: Matching Familiar Figures (MFF), Kagan (1966); Contingency Naming Test (CNT), Anderson et al. (2000); Trail Making Test (A-TM), Reitan (1971); Logan Stop Signal Task (SST), Logan (1994). Goal Setting: Rey-Osterrieth Complex Figure (ROCFT), Rey (1941); Tower of London (TOL), Shallice (1982). Cognitive Flexibility: Controlled Oral Word Association Test (COWAT), Gaddes and Crockett (1975); Contingency Naming Test (CNT: 3and4), Anderson et al. (2000); Concept Generation Test (CGT), Jacobs et al. (2001); Wisconsin Card Sorting Test (WCST), Heaton (1981); Stroop Color Word Test (SCWT), Golden (1978). Executive Batteries: NEPSY, Korkman et al. (1998); BADS-C, Emslie, Wilson, Burden, Nimmo-Smith and Wilson (2003); Preschool EF Battery (PEFB), Espy, Kaufmann, Glisky and McDiarmid (2001); NASAC, Anderson et al. (1995). For a screening evaluation of executive functions it is indicated the use of the Frontal Assessment Battery – FAB (Dubois et al., 2000) and to assess decision-making the best instrument is the Iowa Gambling Task (IGT) (Bechara et al., 1994).

Psychiatric Symptoms Related to TBI in Prefrontal Cortex

Once that the prefrontal cortex, between its many functions, also regulates the behavior, TBI in this area leads to the development of psychiatric symptoms. According to Fay et al. (2012) 36% of the children who had moderated or severe TBI tend to present symptoms compatible to some kind of psychiatric disorder in the 2 years following the injury.

According to McKinlay (2002), TBI in preschool children is associated with persisting negative effects on psychosocial development in adolescence. The study pointed that these children were more likely to develop attention-deficit-hyperactivity disorder (ADHD), conduct disorder, substance abuse and mood disorder. Another study (Andrews, Rose and Johnson, 1998) showed that children who had TBI presented lower self-steem, were lonelier and had higher rates of antisocial behavior. Children who had more severe injuries had more problems at school, were engaged in fewer social activities and reported having fewer friends than the ones with less severe injury (Janusz, Kirkwood,

Yeates and Taylor, 2002; Fletcher, Ewing-Cobbs, Miner, Levin and Eisenberg, 1990).

Mood Disorders: Depression, Mania, Apathy and Emotional Lability

Depression is the most common psychiatric disorder after TBI. Children with left anterior (frontal) lesions are more likely to have depressive symptoms. The majority of children who develop depressed mood following TBI have pre-injury risk factors, such as personal history of depressed mood or parents with a history of mood disorders (Kreutzer, Seel and Gourley, 2001). Still, depressed mood in subjects with no premorbid history of depression were found. It has also been found that TBI may increase the risk of depression, particularly in socially disadvantaged children (Kreutzer, Seel and Gourley, 2001; Vaishnavi, Rao and Fann, 2009).

Research studies suggest a small incidence of mania following TBI. Van Reekum, Cohen and Wong (2000) revised several studies and found that 4.2% of all subjects had the diagnosis of mania directly caused by TBI. Mania disorder following TBI usually presents more aggressive and irritable symptoms and less euphoria. Predisposing factors for development of mania after TBI are damage to the basal region of right temporal lobe and right orbitofrontal cortex and individuals with family history of bipolar disorder (Mustafa, Evrim and Sarı, 2005).

Also, Max et al. (2000) used the Neuropsychiatric Rating Scale in 94 children and adolescents with ages between 5 and 14 and they found mood lability in 49% of the subjects and apathy in 14%.

Anxiety

Overanxious disorders, specific phobias, separation anxiety disorders, and social anxiety disorders reflect the various types of anxiety that children often experience following brain injury. Traumatic brain injury, especially with prefrontal cortex damage, is associated with an increased incidence of anxiety symptoms. The amygdala is central to the development and expression of conditioned fear reactions, and studies in humans and animals have shown that learning to inhibit these fear reactions involves inhibition by the ventral medial prefrontal cortex (Etkin, Egner and Kalisch, 2011). Patients with anxiety symptoms have diminished activation of the ventral medial prefrontal cortex during the processing of fear.

It is possible that a person's capacity to regulate the fear reaction may be impaired after mild traumatic brain injury because the neural networks involved in the regulation of anxiety may be damaged as a result of the traumatic brain injury (Byrant, 2008; 2011; Simmons and Matthews, 2012). TBI also decreases the neurotrophic factor levels such as vascular endothelial growth factor (VEGF) in the PFC which is known as anxiolytic. The change in VEGF levels alters the cell proliferation and maturation in the brain region such as PFC (Baykara et al., 2012).

Substance Abuse, Gambling and Other Compulsive Behavior

Investigations suggest that prefrontal cortex dysfunction may produce impulsive behavior and greater risk for substance use disorders (Chambers, Taylor and Potenza, 2003).

There are also evidences that TBI may increase drug or alcohol use in persons with no histories of significant substance use prior to the injury. Especially if the injury reaches the orbitofrontal cortex (Bjork and Grant, 2009).

Once that TBI in prefrontal cortex has a great impact on executive functions, increased preference for small-immediate rewards over large-delayed rewards is expected (McHugh and Wood, 2008).

In a betting game, subjects who had TBI also made more impulsive choices, and responded suboptimally to changes in reward probability (Salmond and Jacquelyn, 2005). It happens because of the disability in the regulation of motivational behavior, recompenses systems and inhibitory control. This preference for immediate recompense is also observable in individuals addicted to substances, which suggests that people who had TBI, especially those with prefrontal injury, may be impaired in their ability to generate a mental representation of potential long-term negative consequences of drug use, a process also called "*Miopia for the Future*" (Bjork and Grant, 2009; Bechara et al., 1994).

Psychosis

Psychosis secondary to traumatic brain injury is reported to occur in anywhere from 4% to 8.9% of individuals who sustained TBI (Fujii, 2002). McAllister and Ferrell (2000) have noted a connection between the development of psychotic symptoms and orbital frontal, temporal, and basal ganglia damage following TBI.

Although there are evidences that TBI in the prefrontal cortex and psychosis are connected, the significance of this association has not been clarified yet.

Conduct Disorder and Aggressive Behavior

Studies suggest that lesions to the prefrontal cortex early in life are strictly connected to the development of antisocial and aggressive behavior in children and adolescents (Raine, 2002). Pennington and Bennetto (1993) investigated nine cases of children who had frontal lesions in the first 10 years of life. All of the subjects developed behavioral problems, 7 of them being conduct disordered.

TBI AND PROGNOSTIC PREDICTORS

Cognitive reserve and environmental factors are also predictors of the long-term prognosis. Cognitive reserve is a concept that was developed to explain inter-individual variability in the response to brain damage and neurological disorders. Higher preinjury cognitive reserve has been linked to a higher level of intellectual functioning after the injury. Definitions of cognitive reserve have generally used preinjury intellectual level (IQ) to be determined. According to Kirkwood, Yeates, Randolph and Kirk (2012), there are many tests which may evaluate the premorbid IQ of the children/adolescents who had a TBI. The Wechsler Intelligence Scale for Children – Fourth Edition (WISC–IV), is one of the most utilized instruments to evaluate intelligence thought diverse sub-tests, especially those used to evaluate consolidated verbal abilities such as Vocabulary and Information (Lezak et al., 2004). Even when TBI is diffuse or bilateral, Vocabulary tends to be among the least affected of the WISC battery tests (Lezak et al., 2004); Also, the California Verbal Learning Test–Children's Version (CVLT–C) measures verbal learning and memory; The Grooved Pegboard evaluates speed and dexterity of the fine motor coordination; The Woodcock–Johnson III Tests of Achievement (WJ–III), evaluates Reading ability; Word Memory Test (WMT), evaluates evocation ability. Level of education, brain size and academic achievement have all been found to be positively related to prognosis as well (Howieson, Loring and Hannay, 2004)

The best outcomes have been associated to good social support and family cohesion. Genetic characteristics may also play a role in this process, but further studies are necessary to address to what extent the interaction between genetic, premorbid cognitive reserve and environmental factors are crucial for the rehabilitation process.

Outcomes after TBI in children/adolescents are highly variable.

NEUROPLASTICITY AFTER TBI

Studies with animals suggest that the neurochemical environment of the brain after TBI (as well as others brain injuries) becomes more "immature" (Cramer and Chopp, 2000), which facilitates the plasticity occurrence. However, such plasticity is not always functional. The adaptive plasticity after TBI is, usually, the one that happens after relearning and practical action in the remaining neural network (Forsyth and Kirkham, 2012).

RECOVERY STRATEGIES

Neuropsychological Evaluation

Neuropsychology is a specialty of the psychology that studies the structure and function of the central nervous system as it relate to psychological processes and behaviors in both normal and abnormal conditions.

The neuropsychological evaluation is a method that combines investigation about the patient complain and testing. The results may guide the professional to effective treatment methods for the rehabilitation of patients by indicating which cognitive abilities are intact and which ones have been impaired and how impaired they are. A careful Neuropsychological Evaluation is always a very important procedure to investigate cognitive strengthens and weaknesses after TBI, such as whether verbal or visual functions are more depressed, and the extent to which retrieval memory problems, frontal behavioral disinhibition, or impaired executive functioning each contribute to the child poor performance on daily and educational tasks (Hannay, Howieson, Loring, Fischer and Lezak, 2004).

Cognitive Rehabilitation

The goal of the cognitive rehabilitation with TBI patients is to assist the individual in the process of recovering or compensating the damaged cognitive functions so he/she can move through daily life. The restorative approach is focused on reinforcing the functions that remain at least in some extent intact. The compensatory approach focuses on training the patients on new strategies to cope with the impairment (Freire, Coelho, Lacerda, 2011).

The cognitive rehabilitation treatment varies depending on individual deficits. Usually, a neuropsychological evaluation is completed to determine which and how the cognitive functions may be trained before the treatment with cognitive rehabilitation begins.

The treatment involves the training of day life activities and repetitive exercises of writing, drawing and verbal processes.

Family

Successful rehabilitation requires family cooperation in a variety of areas such as transportation, finances, leisure, and emotional support (Jacobs, 1988). Family functioning has been associated with greater improvement in people with TBI, including improvement in overall disability, level of functioning, and employability in the future. The family may be helpful by proposing activities, after they get oriented by professionals and motivating the child/adolescent.

The person with injury may be more vulnerable to environmental stressors that may difficult and also impede the recovery process. Caregiver distress may diminish the effectiveness of rehabilitation.

Unfortunately, there is evidence that family members experience substantial emotional distress and family dysfunction after injury (Sander, Maestas, Sherer, Malec and Richardson, 2012). Parents can also stimulate children with TBI in the prefrontal cortex by encouraging them to play board games, for example. Children and adolescents must be encouraged to exercise as much self-control as possible in the context of enjoyable experiences such as playing, since this activity require them to resist impulses (Aamodt and Wang, 2011). Structured play with other children can also improve executive function, cognitive flexibility and social interaction.

School

Children/adolescents who have physical impairments associated with the TBI are most easily comprehended. When a child/adolescent enters the classroom in a wheelchair, for example, the teachers as well as the other students, are reminded that he has sustained injuries.

On the other hand, when the subject seems healthy, walking and interacting with no obvious physical deficits, which is the case of individuals who had TBI in prefrontal cortex, people tend to assume that he is completely recovered and requires no academic or behavioral assistance.

Educators are not usually prepared to deal with students who had TBI. They currently have a limited behavioral repertory to assist those students once they are back to classroom (Berbaum, 2007). Unfortunately, there are no usual procedures or curricula specifically for students with TBI.

According to Vygotsky (1978) and his concept of Zone of Proximal Development (ZPD), the learning process may be stimulated by an interactive environment, in which the teacher and other students may contribute to the development of cognitive abilities of the learner. The ZPD is, basically, the difference between what a learner can do alone and what he can do with help (Hedegaard, 2005).

According to Shabani, Khatib and Ebadi (2010), the learner may be kept in his own ZPD as often as possible by solving tasks that are slightly harder than what he is able to do by himself. The aim of this process is that, after completing the task with help (sometimes more than once), the individual may be able to do the same thing alone.

When the learner is a child/adolescent who had TBI in prefrontal cortex, the applying of this method is even more important. By working with help, the individual identifies his own potential, which motivates them in the learning process. Besides that, by the repetition, in peers, of activities that require more abilities than he has at the moment, the subjects may adapt skills and develop new ones to complete the activity.

Berbaum (2007) suggests that there are two essential forms to assist the children/adolescents who had TBI in the learning process: adaptation of the learning environment and accommodation of the student impairment.

Adaptation occurs by the use of alternative strategies to evaluate the student academic skills, as well as altering the presentation mode to make the comprehension easier. Accommodation includes modification of demands and expectations for the student according to his/her abilities and competencies in specific skill domains.

Tyler, Blosser, and DePompei (1999) provided a list with common difficulties of children/adolescents who had TBI at school and suggestions about how to deal with it. Concentration/attention: reduce distractions; divide activities in smaller units so the student can complete one section at time; ask the student to review the information that has been presented; create a signaling system to ask the student to pay attention. Memory: regularly repeat and summarize information; orient the student to use devices (calendars, sticky notes, etc) to compensate memory impairments; link the new information with the student's relevant previous knowledge. Organization: provide for the student extra time to review his/her work; checklists of steps for complex tasks.

Pharmacological Strategies

Because of the diversity of symptoms in patients with TBI and the differences in the form that any individual may react to a medication, there is no general pharmacologic treatment for people who had TBI. The individual symptoms must be carefully observed before the treatment is planned.

As it has been said before, TBI in prefrontal cortex may cause neuropsychiatric symptoms, neurocognitive deficits and neurobehavioral impairments. The most commonly medication used in these cases are:

Stimulants

TBI is associated with decreased dopamine activity and stimulants increases extracellular dopamine levels, especially in the frontal cortex.

The most commonly used stimulant by people who had TBI is methylphenidate. The literature reports that it has been safely used in adults and pediatric patients with positive effects on cognitive functions including memory, executive functions, attention and global cognition (Writer and Schillerstrom, 2009; Talsky et al., 2010).

Nonstimulant Dopamine Enhancers (Antiparkinsonian Drugs)

Such as the stimulants, these drugs serve to increase dopamine levels in the brain. It functions as an agonist or dopamine precursor. The most commonly used types are amantadine, bromocriptine, pramipexole and carbidopa (Talsky et al., 2010). Studies reported that nonstimulant dopamine enhancers improve executive functioning, attention, global cognitive functioning, memory and language in adults and pediatric patients who had TBI (Writer and Schillerstrom, 2009).

Acetylcholinesterase Inhibitors

Acetylcholinesterase inhibitors increase the acetylcholine levels restoring regular cholinergic synaptic transmission, which is impaired by TBI. Studies (Zhang, Plotkin and Wang, 2004; Tenovuo, 2005) related that acetylcholinesterase inhibitors do have a positive impact on neurocognitive abilities of patients who had TBI, notably in memory and attention.

Mood Stabilizers (Anticonvulsants)

This class of medications embraces drugs such as valproic acid, carbamazepine, lamotrigine, oxcarbazepine. These anticonvulsants are used in the treatment of violent behaviors, bipolar symptomatology, manic symptoms, lability of mood.

They may be useful in the treatment of neuropsychiatric symptoms of TBI patients, but their impact in cognitive skills is controversy (Talsky et al., 2010). Smith, et al. (1994) reported that long-term carbamazepine use in TBI adults and pediatric patients had negative effects on cognition including executive functioning, sensory-motor-perceptual skills, and attention. Other studies (Chatham-Showalter and Kimmel, 2000; Dikmen et al., 2000) pointed that valproic acid have positive neurocognitive effects including improved recent memory and problem-solving, but also have negative impact on decision making speed.

Antidepressants

Evidences suggest that antidepressant can be useful on the treatment of both neuropsychiatric and neurocognitive deficits persisting from TBI (Talsky et al., 2010).

The uses of selective serotonin reuptake inhibitors (SSRIs) have shown improve on behavior, neurocognitive and neuropsychiatric deficits, particularly agitation, depression, psychomotor retardation and recent memory lost (Writer and Schillerstrom, 2009).

Conclusion

The neuropsychological consequences of TBI in prefrontal cortex during childhood/adolescence are very complex and depends on a variety of factors. All the valid strategies to be adopted after TBI must include an integration of behavioral, familiar, educational and pharmacological approaches, that may contribute to a shorter recovery time of the young people in development. There are promising treatments with stimulant drugs and neuropsychological rehabilitation, but further studies are required to define to what extent individuals affected by TBI may have a complete restoration (or not) of premorbid cognitive abilities by making use of these integrated techniques.

Acknowledgments

Dr. Paulo Jannuzzi Cunha would like to thank FAPESP (Grant 2010/ 15604-0).

References

Aamodt, S., Wang, S. (2011). Welcome to your child´s brain: How the mind grows from conception to college. New York: Ed. Bloomsburry.

Anderson, C. V., Bigler, E. D, Blatter, D. D. (1995). Frontal lobe lesions, diffuse damage, and neuropsychological functioning in traumatic brain-injured patients. *Journal of Clinical and Experimental Neuropsychology*, 17(6), pp. 900-908.

Anderson, P., Anderson V., Northam, E., Taylor, H. G. (2000). Standardization of the Contingency Naming Test for school-aged children: a new measure of reactive flexibility. *Clinical Neuropsychological Assesment,* 1, pp. 247-273.

Anderson, V., Godfrey, C., Rosenfeld, J. V., Catroppa, C. (2012). 10 years outcome from childhood traumatic brain injury. *Internacional Journal of Developmental Neuroscience*, 30, pp. 217-224.

Anderson, V. A., Brown, S., Newitt, H. (2010). What Contributes to Quality of Life in Adult Survivors of Childhood Traumatic Brain Injury?. *Journal of Neurotrauma,* 27, pp. 863-870.

Anderson, V. A. et al. (1997). Predicting recovery from head injury in young children: A prospective analysis. *Journal of the International Neuropsychological Society*, 3, pp. 568-580.

Andrews, T. K., Rose, F. D., Johnson, D. A. (1998). Social and behavioral effects of traumatic brain injury in children. *Brain Injury*, 12, pp. 133-138.

Arciniegas, D. B., Anderson, C. A., Topkoff, J., McAllister, T. W. (2005). Mild traumatic brain injury: a neuropsychiatric approach to diagnosis, evaluation, and treatment. *Neuropsychiatric Disease and Treatment*, 1(4), pp. 311-327.

Baykara, B., et al. (2012). Anxiety Caused by Traumatic Brain Injury Correlates to Decreased Prefrontal Cortex Vegf Immunoreactivity and Neuron Density in Immature Rats. *Turkish Neurosurgery*, 22(5), pp. 604-610.

Bechara, A., Damasio, A. R., Damasio, H., Anderson, S. W. (1994). Insensitivity to future consequences following damage to human prefrontal cortex. *Cognition*, 50, pp. 7-15.

Berbaum, C. (2007). School Reintegration Following Traumatic Brain Injury in Children and Adolescents. Dissertation Abstracts International Section A: Humanities and Social Sciences, Walden University.

Bjork, J. M., Grant, S. J. (2009). Does Traumatic Brain Injury Increase Risk for Substance Abuse?. *Journal of Neurotrauma*, 26(7), pp. 1077-1082.

Blackmore, S. J. (2008). Special Issue: Neurocognitive Approaches to Developmental Disorders: A Festschrift for Uta Frith. *The Quarterly Journal of Experimental Psychology,* 61(1), pp. 40-49.

Blackmore, S. J. (2011). Imaging brain development: The adolescent brain. *Neuroimage*, 61(2), pp. 397-406.

Blackmore, S. J., Burnett, S., Dahl, R. E. (2010). The role of puberty in the developing adolescent brain. *Human Brain Mapping*, 31(6), pp. 926-933.

Bruer, J. T. (1998). The brain and child development: time for some critical thinking. *Public Health Reports*, 113, pp. 388-397.

Byrant, R. A. (2008). Disentangling mild traumatic brain injury and stress reactions. *Journal of Traumatic Stress*, 9(3), pp. 621-629.

Byrant, R. A. (2011). Post-traumatic stress disorder vs traumatic brain injury. *Dialogues in Clinical Neurosciense*. 13(3), pp. 251-262.

Chambers, R. A., Taylor, J. R., Potenza, M. N. (2003). Developmental Neurocircuitry of Motivation in Adolescence: A Critical Period of Addiction Vulnerability. *American Journal of Psychiatry*, 160(6), pp. 1041-1052.

Chan, R. C. K., Shum, D., Toulopoulou, T., Chen, E. Y. H. (2008). Assessment of executive functions: Review of instruments and identification of critical issues. *Archives of Clinical Neuropsychology*, 23, pp. 201-216.

Chatham-Showalter, P., Kimmel, D. N. (2000) Agitated symptom response to divalproex following acute brain injury. *Journal Neuropsychiatry Clinical Neuroscience*, 12, pp. 395-397.

Cicchetti, D., Curtis, W. J. (2006). The Developing Brain and Neural Plasticity: Implications for Normality, Psychopathology, and Resilience. In: Developmental Psychopathology: *Developmental Neuroscience* (Vol. 2) (pp. 1-64). New York: Wiley.

Cramer, S. C., Chopp, M. (2000). Recovery recapitulates ontogeny. *Trends Neuroscience,* 23, pp. 265-71.

Dennis, M. (2010). Margaret Kennard (1899–1975): Not a 'Principle' of Brain Plasticity but a Founding Mother of Developmental Neuropsychology. *Cortex*, 46(8), pp. 1043-1059.

Dikmen, S., et al. (2000). Neuropsychological effects of valproate in traumatic brain injury. *Neurology*, 54, pp. 895-902.

Dikmen, S. S., et al. (2009). Cognitive Outcome Following Traumatic Brain Injury. *Journal of Head Trauma Rehabilitation*, 24(6), pp. 430-438.

Dubois, B., et al. Slachevsky, A., Litvan, I., Pillon, B. (2000). The FAB: a Frontal Assessment Battery at bedside. *Neurology*, 55(11), pp. 1621-1626.

Emslie, H., Wilson, F. C., Burden, V., Nimmo-Smith, I., and Wilson, B. A. (2003) Behavioural Assessment of the Dysexecutive Syndrome for Children (BADS-C). *Child Neuropsychology,* 13, pp. 539-542.

Epsy, K. A., Kaufmann, P. M., McDiarmid, M. D., Glisky, M. L. (2001). New procedures to access executive functions in preschool children. *The Clinical Neuropsychologist,* 15(1), pp. 46-58.

Etkin, A., Egner, T., Kalisch, R. (2011). Emotional processing in anterior cingulate and medial prefrontal cortex. *Trends in Cognitive Sciences*, 15(9), pp. 85-93.

Ewing-Cobbs, L., Bloom, D. R. (1999). Traumatic Brain Injury (pp. 262-288). In: Brown, R. T. *Cognitive aspects of chronic illness in children*. NY: The Guilford Press.

Fay, G. C., Jaffe, K. M., Polissar, N. L., Liao, S., Rivara, J. B., Martin, K.M. (1994). Outcome of pediatric traumatic brain injury at three years: A cohort study. *Archives of Physical Medicine and Rehabilitation*, 75, pp. 733-741.

Fay, T. B., Yeates, K. O., Wade, S. L., Drotar, D., Stancin, T., Taylor, H. G. (2009). Predicting longitudinal patterns of functional deficits in children with traumatic brain injury. *Neuropsychology*, 23(3), pp. 271-282.

Fletcher, J. M., Ewing-Cobbs, L., Miner, M. E., Levin, H. S., Eisenberg, H. M. (1990). Behavioral changes after closed head injury in children. *Journal of Consulting and Clinical Psychology*, 58(1), pp. 93-98.

Fonseca, R., Zimmermann, N., Cotrena, C., Cardoso, C., Kristensen, C. H., Grassi-Oliveira, R. (2012). Neuropsychological assessment of executive functions in traumatic brain injury: hot and cold components. *Psychology and Neuroscience*, 5(2), pp.183-190.

Forsyth, R., Kirkham, F. (2012). Predicting outcome after childhood brain injury. *Canadian Medical Association or its licensors*, 184(11), pp. 1257-1264.

Freire, F. R., et al. (2011). Cognitive rehabilitation following traumatic brain injury. *Dementia and Neuropsychologia*, 5(1), pp.17-25.

Fujii, D. (2002). Neuropsychiatry of Psychosis Secondary to Traumatic Brain Injury. *Psychiatric Times*, 19(8), pp. 1-2.

Gaddes, W. H., Crockett, D. J. (1975). The Spreen Benton Aphasia Tests: Normative data as a measure of normal language development. *Brain and Language*, 2, pp. 257-279.

García-Molina, A., Ensenat-Cantallops, A, Tirapu-Ustarroz, J., Roig-Rovira, T. (2009). Maduración de la corteza prefrontal y desarrollo de las funciones ejecutivas durante los primeros cinco años de vida. *Revista de Neurología,* 48(8), pp. 435-440.

Gogtay, N., et al. (2004). Dynamic mapping of human cortical development during childhood through early adulthood. *PNAS*, 101(21), pp. 8174-8179.

Golden, C. J. (1978). *Stroop color and word test: A manual for clinical and experimental users* (pp.1-32). Chicago: Skoelting Company.

Hannay, H. J., Howieson, D. B., Loring, D. W., Fischer, J. S., Lezak, M. D. (2004). Neuropathology for Neuropsychologists. In: Lezak, M. D., Howieson, D. B., Loring, D. W. (Org.), *Neuropsychological Assessment* (pp. 157-285). New York: Oxford University Press.

Heaton, R. (1981). *A manual for the Wisconsin Card Sorting Test*. Florida: Psychological Assesment Resources.

Hedegaard, M. (2005). The zone of proximal development as basis for instruction (pp. 225-284). In: Daniels, H. *An introduction to Vygotsky*. US: Ed. Routledge.

Howieson, D. B., Loring, D. W., Hannay, H. J. (2004). Neurobehavioral Variables and Diagnostic Issues. In: Lezak, M. D., Howieson, D. B., Loring, D. W. (Org.), *Neuropsychological Assessment* (pp. 286-336). New York: Oxford University Press.

Jacobs, R., Anderson, V., Harvey, A. S. (2001). Concept Generation Test: A measure of conceptual reasoning skills in children. Examination of developmental trends. *Clinical Neuropsychological Assessment*, 2, pp. 101-117.

Jacobs, H. E. (1988). Vocational rehabilitation (pp. 245-284). In: Liberman, R. P. *Psychiatn'c Rehabilitation of Chronic Mental* Patients. Washington, DC: American Psychiatric Press.

Janusz, J. A., Kirkwood, M. W., Yeates, K. O., Taylor, H. G. (2002). Social problem-solving skills in children with traumatic brain injury: long-term outcomes and prediction of social competence. *Child Neuropsychology*, 8, pp. 179-94.

Johnson, M. H. (2001) Functional brain development in humans. Nature reviews *Neuroscience*, 2, pp. 475-483.

Kagan, J. (1966). Reflection-impulsity: The generality and dynamics of conceptual temp. *Journal of Abnormal Psychology*, 71, pp. 75-81.

Kalia, M. (2008). Brain development: anatomy, connectivity, adaptive plasticity, and toxicity. *Metabolism*, 57(2), pp. S2-S5.

Kirkwood, M. W., Yeates, K. O., Randolph, C. K., Kirk, J. W. (2012). The implications of symptom validity test failure for ability-based test performance in a pediatric sample. *Psychological Assessment*,24(1), pp. 36-45.

Koehler, R., Wilhem, E., Shoulson, I. (2011). *Cognitive Rehabilitation Therapy for Traumatic Brain Injury: Evaluating the Evidence*. Institute of Medicine of the National Academies. Washington: The National Academies Press. pp. 1-272.

Kolb, B., Gibb, R., Gorny, G. (2000). Cortical plasticity and the development of behavior after early frontal cortical injury. *Developmental Neuropsychology*, 18, pp. 423-44.

Korkman, M., Kirk, U., Kemp S. (1998). *NEPSY-A Developmental Neuropsychological Assessment*. Texas: The Psychological Corporation.

Kreutzer, J. S., Seel, R. T., Gourley, E. (2001). The prevalence and symptom rates of depression after traumatic brain injury: a comprehensive examination. *Brain Injury*, 15 (7), pp. 563-576.

Lezak, M. D., Howieson, D. B., Loring, D. W. (2004). *Neuropsychological Assessment* – Fourth Edition. New York: Oxford University Press.

Logan, G. D. (1994). On the ability to inhibit thought and action: A users guide to the stop-signal paradigm. In: Dagenbach, D., Carr, T. H. *Inhibitory processes in attention, memory, and language*. (pp. 189–239). San Diego: Academic Press.

Lovell, M. R., Franzen, M. D. (1994). Neuropsychological Assessment. In: Silver, J. M., Yudofsky, S. C., Hales, R. E. (Org.), *Neuropsychiatry of traumatic brain injury*. (pp. 133-160). American Psychiatric Press.

Luria, A. R. (1973). *The Working brain: An introduction to neuropsychology*. New York: Basic.

Max, J. E., et al. (1998). Traumatic Brain Injury in Children and Adolescents: Psychiatric Disorders at Two Years. *Journal of the American Academy of Child and Adolescent Psychiatry*, 36(9), pp.1278-1285.

Max, J. E., et al. (2000). Personality change disorder in children and adolescents following traumatic brain injury. *Journal of International Neuropsychological Society*, 6(3), pp. 279-289.

McAllister, T. W., Ferrell, R. B. (2000). Evaluation and treatment of psychosis after traumatic brain injury. *NeuroRehabilitation*, 17, pp. 357-368.

McHugh., L., Wood, R. L. (2008) Using a temporal discounting paradigm to measure decision-making and impulsivity following traumatic brain injury: a pilot study. *Brain Inj.*, 22, pp. 715–721.

McKinlay, A., Grace, R. C., Horwood, L. J., Fergusson, D. M., MacFarlane, M. R. (2010). Long-term behavioural outcomes of pre-school mild traumatic brain injury. *Child: Care, Health and Development*, 36, pp. 22-30.

Mustafa, B., Evrim, O., Sari, A. (2005). Secondary Mania Following Traumatic Brain Injury. *The Journal of Neuropsychiatry and Clinical Neurosciences,* 17(1), pp.122-124.

Pennington, B. F., Bennetto, L. (1993). Main effects or transactions in the neuropsychology of conduct disorder? Commentary on "The neuropsychology of conduct disorder". *Development and Psychopathology,* 5, pp. 153–164.

Raine, A. (2002). Annotation: The role of prefrontal deficits, low autonomic arousal, and early health factors in the development of antisocial and aggressive behavior in children. *Journal of Child Psychology and Psychiatry,* 43(4), pp. 417-434.

Reitan, R. M. (1971). Trail Making Test Results for Normal and Brain-Damaged Children. *Perceptual and Motor Skills*, 33, pp. 575-581.

Rey, A. (1941). Psychological examination of traumatic encephalopathy. *Archives de Psychologie*, 28, pp. 286–340.

Reznick, J. S, Morrow, J. D., Goldman, B. D., Snyder, J. (2004). The onset of working memory in infants. *Infancy*, 6, pp. 145-54.

Salmond, C. H., Jacquelyn, S. B. (2005). Cognitive outcome in traumatic brain injury survivors. *Neuroscience*, 11(2), pp.111-116.

Sander, A. M., Maestas, K. L., Sherer, M., Malec, J. F., Richardson, R. N. (2012). Relationship of Caregiver and Family Functioning to Participation Outcomes After Postacute Rehabilitation for Traumatic Brain Injury: A Multicenter Investigation. *Archives of Physical Medicine and Rehabilitation,* 93, pp. 842-848.

Shabani, K., Khatib, M., Ebadi, S. (2010) Vygotsky's Zone of Proximal Development: Instructional Implications and Teachers' Professional Development. *Canadian Center of Science and Education*, 3(4), pp.237-248.

Shallice T. (1982). Specific impairments of planning. *Philosophical Transactions of the Royal Society London,* 298, pp. 199–209.

Smith, J. R., K. R., et al. (1994). Neurobehavioral effects of phenytoin and carbamazepine in patients recovering from brain trauma: a comparative study. *Archives of Neurology*, 51, pp. 653–660.

Simmons, A. N., Matthews, S. C. (2012). Neural circuitry of PTSD with or without mild traumatic brain injury: A meta-analysis. *Neuropharmacology*, 62, pp. 598-606.

Stancin, T., et al. (2002). Health-Related Quality of Life of Children and Adolescents After Traumatic Brain Injury. *Pediatrics*, 109, pp. 34

Talsky, A., et al. (2010). Pharmacological interventions for traumatic brain injury. *British Columbia Medical Journal*, 53(1), p. 1.

Tenovuo, O. (2005). Central acetylcholinesterase inhibitors in the treatment of chronic traumatic brain injury-clinical experience in 111 patients. *Progress in Neuropsychopharmacology and Biological Psychiatry,* 29(1), pp. 61-67.

Thompson, N. M., et al. (1994). Motor, visuo-spatial, and somatosensory skills after closed head injury in children and adolescents: A study of change. *Neuropsychology*, 8, pp. 333–342.

Tsuchida, A., Fellows, L. K. (2009). Lesion evidence that two distinct regions within prefrontal cortex are critical for n-back performance in humans. *Neuroscience*, 21, pp. 2263–2275.

Tyler, J., Blosser, J., Depompei, R. (1999). *Teaching Strategies for Students with Brain Injuries.* Wake Forest, NC: Lash and Associates Publishing/ Training Inc.

Vaishnavi, S., Rao, V., Fann, J. R. (2009). Neuropsychiatric Problems After Traumatic Brain Injury: Unraveling the Silent Epidemic. *Psychosomatics*, 50 (3), pp. 198-205.

Van Reekum, R., Cohen, T., Wong, J. (2000). Can traumatic brain injury cause psychiatric disorders? *The Journal of Neuropsychiatry and Clinical Neurosciences,* 12, pp. 316-327.

Vygotsky, L. S. (1978). *Mind in society: The development of higher psychological processes.* Cambridge, MA: Harvard University Press.

Voytek, B., Knight, R. T. (2010). Prefrontal cortex and basal ganglia contributions to visual working memory. *Proceedings of the National Academy of Sciences of the United States of America*, 107, pp. 18167–18172.

Writer, B. W., Schillerstrom, J. E. (2009). Psychopharmacological Treatment for Cognitive Impairment in Survivors of Traumatic Brain Injury: A Critical Review. *The Journal of Neuropsychiatry and Clinical Neurosciences,* 21, pp. 362-370.

Zhang, L., Plotkin, R. C., Wang, G., Sandel, M. E., Lee, S. (2004). Cholinergic augmentation with donepezil enhances recovery in short term memory and sustained attention after traumatic brain injury. *Archives of Physical Medicine and Rehabilitation,* 85, pp. 1050–1055.

In: Prefrontal Cortex
Editors: R. O. Collins and J. L. Adams
ISBN 978-1-62618-663-7

Chapter 5

DEVELOPMENTAL RELATIONSHIP BETWEEN EXECUTIVE FUNCTION AND THE PREFRONTAL CORTEX IN YOUNG CHILDREN

Yusuke Moriguchi[1,*] and Kazuo Hiraki[2]
[1]Department of School Education,
Joetsu University of Education, Joetsu, Japan
[2]Department of Systems Science, University of Tokyo, Tokyo, Japan

ABSTRACT

Executive function refers to the ability to plan and execute task-relevant actions and to inhibit irrelevant actions for the attainment of a specific goal. Extensive adult neuroimaging research has revealed that the lateral prefrontal cortex plays an important role in executive function. Recently, developmental studies have shown behavioral evidence that executive function changes significantly during preschool years. It has been proposed that the maturation of the prefrontal cortex plays an essential role in the development of executive function. However, there is little evidence to support this proposal. We have used near-infrared spectroscopy to examine the relationship between the development of

* Correspondence should be addressed to Yusuke Moriguchi, Joestsu University of Education, 1 Yamayashiki-machi, Joetsu 943-8512, Japan. E-mail: moriguchi@ juen.ac.jp. Tel/Fax: +81-25-521-3415.

executive function and the lateral prefrontal cortex. In this article, we show how the development of executive function is related to the lateral prefrontal cortex from the perspective of developmental cognitive neuroscience. Four studies examined the relationship between executive function and the prefrontal cortex in young children. First, we showed that prefrontal activation correlated with performance on executive function tasks in young children with the Dimensional Change Card Sort (DCCS). Second, we investigated the longitudinal relationship between the prefrontal cortex and executive function in young children and found that children showed better behavioral performance and significantly stronger inferior prefrontal activation at 4 years of age than they did at 3 years of age. Moreover, we demonstrated individual differences in the development of prefrontal activation. Third, we revealed that the prefrontal cortex was activated differently depending on task demands. Fourth, we compared the behavioral and neural responses in typically developing children to children with autism and found that children with autism showed decreased behavioral performances and less activation in the prefrontal area during the DCCS task than typically developing children did. Taken together, these results suggested that the development of executive function might be strongly related to the prefrontal cortex in preschool-aged children. These results contribute to our general understanding of the pathway of cognitive development during early childhood and may lead to the support of and interventions for children with developmental disorders.

Executive function (EF) refers to the higher-order cognitive control process ability both to plan, execute, and monitor appropriate and relevant actions and to inhibit irrelevant and inappropriate actions for the attainment of a specific goal. According to recent theories, EF is not unitary. Instead, it has been proposed that EF has several subcomponents. One influential model has been developed by Miyake and his colleagues (Miyake et al., 2000). They used multiple tasks to measure each EF component and adopted a latent variables approach to extract the variance that was common to those tasks. Miyake et al. (2000) have shown that the 3 major components of EF, Inhibition, Shifting, and Updating (Working Memory), are separable even though they are moderately correlated. Although their studies focused on healthy adult populations, follow-up studies of school-aged children partly confirmed Miyake's findings (Huizinga, Dolan, and van der Molen, 2006; Lehto, Juujarvi, Kooistra, and Pulkkinen, 2003). However, there are still controversies of the data for preschool-aged children. Theoretically, there might be 3 components of EF in young children (Garon, Bryson, and Smith,

2008; Oh and Lewis, 2008), but, empirically, a single-factor model (general EF) has been sufficient to account for the data in preschool-aged children (Wiebe, Espy, and Charak, 2008). In this regard, recently, the importance of the general factor has also been emphasized in adult research. Miyake and colleagues have proposed the unitary/diversity framework of EF, in which Shifting, Updating, and the Common EF factor have been detected (Miyake and Friedman, 2012). Thus, the general EF factor may be relatively important in young children, after which other components may gradually emerge.

Behavioral Evidence of EF in Young Children

It has been repeatedly reported that EF rapidly develops during preschool years at the behavioral level. Several tasks have been used to assess EF in young children (Carlson, 2005). One widely used task is the Stroop-like Day-Night task and Black-White task (Gerstadt, Hong, and Diamond, 1994; Moriguchi, 2012; Simpson and Riggs, 2005). In the Day-Night task, children are instructed to say day in response to a picture of a moon with some stars and night in response to a picture of a sun. In order to perform the task correctly, children have to inhibit a dominant response (e.g., children have to inhibit day responses when presented with a sun card). Response accuracy and response latency improved between 3 and 5 years of age. Although it has been suggested that both inhibition skills and working memory are needed to pass the task, this task is often used as an index of inhibition skills (Carlson and Moses, 2001).

The other task that has been used to index the development of EF is the Dimensional Change Card Sort (DCCS) task (Kirkham, Cruess, and Diamond, 2003; Moriguchi, Lee, and Itakura, 2007; Zelazo, Frye, and Rapus, 1996). In this task, children are asked to sort cards that have 2 dimensions, such as color and shape (e.g., red boats, blue rabbits). There are 2 phases in the task. In the preswitch phase, children are asked to sort cards according to 1 dimension (e.g., color) for several trials. In the postswitch phase, children are asked to sort the cards according to the other dimension (e.g., shape) for several trials. Typically, most 3-year-olds correctly perform the preswitch phase but show difficulty with the postswitch phase. Even though they were asked to sort the cards according to the second dimension, they perseverate to the first dimension. Four- and 5-year-old children correctly sort the cards according to the second dimension. It is highly controversial as to why younger preschoolers exhibit difficulty in the DCCS task. Zelazo and his colleagues have suggested that the younger preschoolers' difficulty in the DCCS stems from difficulty with representing a higher-order rule that integrates 2 incompatible pairs of rules (Zelazo, Muller, Frye, and Marcovitch, 2003). Representing the higher-order rule may improve children's performances in the DCCS tasks. Other researchers have suggested that the failure to inhibit attention to the dimension that was focused on in the preswitch phase may explain 3-year-old children's difficulty in switching to a new dimension in the postswitch phase (Kirkham et al., 2003). Although there has been remaining controversy, the DCCS is used to index cognitive shifting as well as executive function in general (Garon et al., 2008).

There are other tasks that assess the development of EF in preschool-aged children, such as a tapping task (Diamond and Taylor, 1996), a Go/No-go task (Simpson and Riggs, 2007), and a flanker task (Rueda, Rothbart, McCandliss, Saccomanno, and Posner, 2005). In each task, children's performances have been shown to significantly improve during preschool years (Carlson, 2005). Taken together, the behavioral studies strongly suggest that the preschool period is important for the development of EF.

Neural Basis of EF in Young Children

Although the behavioral evidence is accumulating, the neural basis of EF in young children is still unknown. The present article addressed the issue in light of the development of cognitive shifting. It is well known that the prefrontal cortex is a brain region that subserves complex cognitive functions, such as cognitive shifting (Crone, Donohue, Honomichl, Wendelken, and Bunge, 2006). Brain imaging studies have shown that adult participants recruit inferior and dorsolateral prefrontal regions during cognitive shifting tasks, such as the Wisconsin Card Sorting Test (WCST) (Konishi et al., 1998; Monchi, Petrides, Petre, Worsley, and Dagher, 2001). In this task, participants are asked to sort cards depicting geometric features, such as shape, color, and number, according to rules that are detected through feedback from an experimenter. After the participants discover the rule and sort the cards according to that rule for several trials, the rule suddenly changes and the participants must adjust to the rule change depending on the feedback. In this task, participants recruit the prefrontal areas, as well as the parietal cortex, when they have to switch the rules (Konishi et al., 1998; Monchi et al., 2001).

There is some anatomical evidence that the prefrontal cortex develops during the preschool years (Diamond, 2002). Recent structural magnetic resonance imaging (MRI) studies have shown changes in brain structure over time within an individual. Studies by Giedd and colleagues (1999, 2004) have indicated that gray matter in the prefrontal cortex increases in volume during childhood, including the preschool years. Tsujimoto (2008) has suggested that the changes in gray matter volume may imply that the formation of neuronal circuits occurs in the prefrontal cortex during preschool years. Additionally, Giedd and colleagues (1999) have shown that the white matter volume in the frontal area increases linearly during the ages of 4–20 years. Given this evidence, there should be structural changes within the prefrontal cortex during the preschool years.

However, little neuroimaging data have demonstrated the functional development of the prefrontal cortex during the preschool years. Thus, it is still unclear whether the functional development of the prefrontal cortex is associated with significant changes in cognitive shifting in young children. Therefore, we have examined whether inferior prefrontal activation is developmentally correlated with cognitive shifting in young children (Moriguchi and Hiraki, 2009). We have used a near-infrared spectroscopy (NIRS) technique to monitor cerebral hemodynamics by measuring changes in the attenuation of near-infrared light passing through the tissue (Ozonoff, Strayer, McMahon, and Filloux, 1994). Because NIRS is noninvasive and does not require fixing of the body as in functional MRI (fMRI), it is often used for brain imaging studies in infants and children (Matsuda and Hiraki, 2006).

Three-year-old children, 5-year-old children, and adults participated in the study. They were asked to perform the DCCS task, and the brain activation during the DCCS task was examined with a multichannel NIRS system that covered the inferior prefrontal regions that correspond to F7/8 in the International 10/20 system (Okamoto et al., 2004) (Figure 1). We measured changes in the hemoglobin concentrations and its oxygenation levels (oxy-Hb) in the inferior prefrontal areas because the concentration of oxy-Hb has been found to be very sensitive to changes in regional cerebral blood flow. In addition, oxy-Hb provided the strongest correlation with blood-oxygen-level-dependent signals (Strangman, Culver, Thompson, and Boas, 2002). We separately analyzed brain activation during the preswitch and postswitch phases. The brain activation during each phase was compared to the activation during the control phases (adults were instructed to sit still and children were asked to sort blank cards into an extra tray).

At the behavioral level, 5-year-old children and adult participants performed easily during both the preswitch and postswitch phases. Some 3-year-old children performed the DCCS tasks perfectly, but other 3-year-old children committed perseverative errors during the postswitch phases. At the neural level, we observed significant increases in oxy-Hb in the right and left inferior prefrontal areas during the preswitch and postswitch phases compared to the control phase in adults and 5-year-old children. We analyzed the 3-year-old children separately according to whether they committed perseverative errors during the tasks. In the children who did not perseverate (pass group; Figure 2A and 2B), significant oxy-Hb increases were observed in the right inferior prefrontal areas during the preswitch phase and postswitch phases compared to the control phase. In contrast, children who perseverated (perseverate group) exhibited no significant oxy-Hb increases in either the right or left inferior prefrontal areas during both the preswitch and postswitch phases (Figure 3A and 3B). We directly compared the changes in oxy-Hb in the inferior prefrontal regions in the perseverate group to those in the pass group. The results revealed that children in the pass group exhibited greater changes in oxy-Hb in both the right and left inferior prefrontal areas during the preswitch phase and in the right inferior prefrontal areas during the postswitch phase than those in the perseverate group.

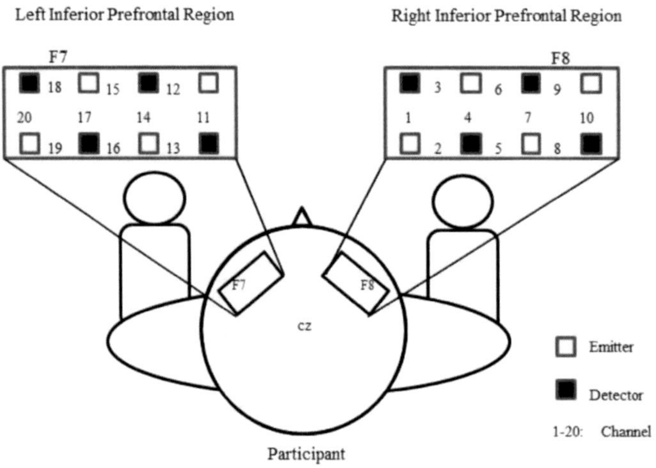

Figure 1. The near-infrared spectroscopy (NIRS) probe was attached to the inferior prefrontal area. Each channel consisted of 1 emitter optode and 1 detector optode.

The differences between the children in the pass group and those in the perseverate group were associated with activation of the right inferior prefrontal cortex during both the preswitch and postswitch phases. Given the differences, it is likely that sustained right inferior prefrontal activation across the preswitch and postswitch phases may be responsible for the development of cognitive shifting during the DCCS task. In order to confirm this issue, we conducted a longitudinal study of children in the pass group and in the perseverate group.

LONGITUDINAL RESEARCH ON THE DEVELOPMENT OF PREFRONTAL FUNCTION IN YOUNG CHILDREN

Most neuroimaging studies in children have relied on a cross-sectional design in which an investigator observes several age groups simultaneously. Cross-sectional research can clarify differences in brain activation and cognitive performance between 2 different age groups, but it cannot address how the differences occur. Therefore, longitudinal approaches are needed to address these issues. To that end, we conducted a longitudinal study of the development of prefrontal function (Moriguchi and Hiraki, 2011). We recruited the children who were involved in the first study again after 1 year. Children were asked to perform the DCCS task, and developmental changes in prefrontal activation were examined with a NIRS technique at 3 years of age (Time 1) and at 4 years of age (Time 2). The procedure and apparatus were the same at Time 1 and Time 2 except for the stimuli used (cards).

As a result, behaviorally, children in the perseverate group (i.e., the children who committed errors at Time 1) improved their performances significantly. None of the children committed perseverative errors at Time 2. In addition, children in the pass group (i.e., the children who did not commit errors at Time 1) performed correctly at Time 2. Thus, there were no significant behavioral differences between the children in the pass group and the perseverate group at Time 2.

Next, we examined whether children showed similar or different brain activations at Time 1 and Time 2. First, children in the pass group showed significant right inferior prefrontal activation during the preswitch and postswitch phases at Time 1 and Time 2, and they significantly activated the left inferior prefrontal areas during the preswitch and postswitch phases at Time 2 compared to Time 1 (Figure 2A, 2B, 2C and 2D). These results revealed that children in the pass group exhibited right inferior prefrontal activation at Time 1, whereas they exhibited bilateral inferior prefrontal activation at Time 2. The activation pattern at Time 2 was similar to that found in 5-year-old children in the first study who exhibited bilateral inferior prefrontal activation during the DCCS task. It is likely that a developmental process exists where children first engage the right inferior prefrontal regions and then recruit the right and left inferior prefrontal regions during the DCCS task.

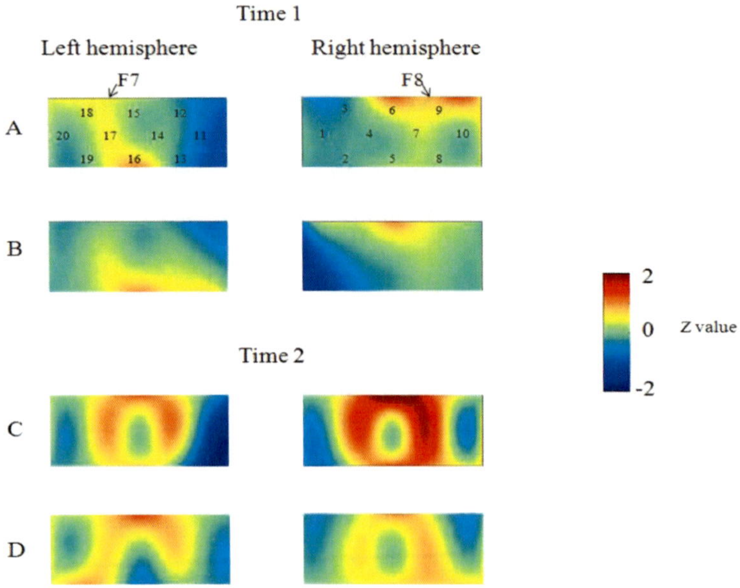

Figure 2. The brain activations of children in the pass group at the first study (Time 1) (AB) and the second study (Time 2) (CD). The grand averaged data during the task phases over the control phases are shown. The numbers (1–10) indicate the channel of the NIRS probe. (A) and (C) show the brain activations during the preswitch phases, and (B) and (D) show the brain activations during the postswitch phases. The red areas highlight areas where stronger activations were observed during the task, and the blue areas highlight areas where deactivations were observed during the task. Figure from Moriguchi, Y., & Hiraki, K. (2011). Longitudinal development of prefrontal function during early childhood. *Developmental Cognitive Neuroscience*, 1, 153-162., with permission from Elsevier.

However, the results in the perseverate group showed a different pattern (Figure 3C and 3D). At Time 1, children in the perseverate group exhibited no significant oxy-Hb increases in either the right or left inferior prefrontal areas during the task phases compared to the control phases. However, at Time 2, they showed significant increases in oxy-Hb in the left (but not right) inferior prefrontal regions during the preswitch and postswitch phases compared to the control phases. We directly compared the brain activations at Time 1 with those at Time 2 and found that children in the perseverate group significantly improved activation in the left inferior prefrontal areas during the preswitch phase and the postswitch phase at Time 2 compared to Time 1. These results revealed that children in the perseverate group exhibited no significant inferior prefrontal activation at Time 1, but they showed significant left inferior prefrontal activation at Time 2 during the DCCS tasks.

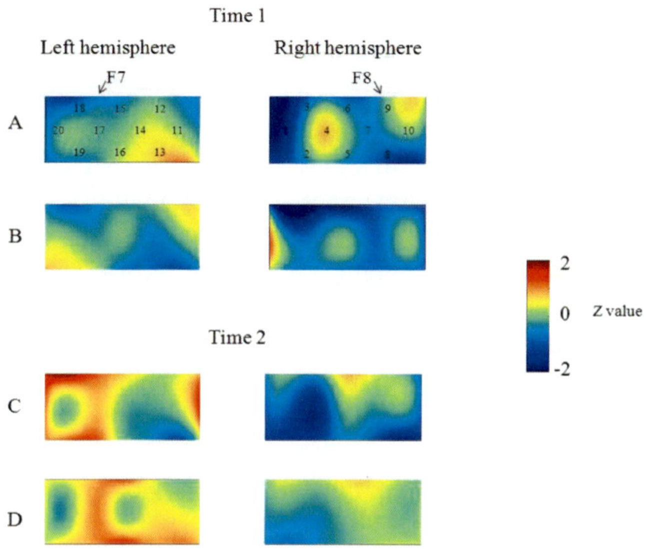

Figure 3. The brain activations of children in the perseverate groupat the first study (Time 1) (AB) and the second study (Time 2) (CD). The grand averaged data during the task phases over the control phases are shown. The numbers (1–10) indicate the channel of the NIRS probe. (A) and (C) show the brain activations during the preswitch phases, and (B) and (D) show the brain activations during the postswitch phases. The red areas highlight areas where stronger activations were observed during the task, and the blue areas highlight areas where deactivations were observed during the task. Figure from Moriguchi, Y., & Hiraki, K. (2011). Longitudinal development of prefrontal function during early childhood. *Developmental Cognitive Neuroscience*, 1, 153-162., with permission from Elsevier.

Two important results emerged when we combined the first and second studies. First, sustained unilateral (either right or left) inferior prefrontal activation across the preswitch and postswitch phases may be important for successful performance in the DCCS task. That is, it seems likely that activation in the inferior prefrontal regions is important in the postswitch phases, but our results did not support that idea. Similar results were obtained in an event-related potential study of DCCS (Espinet, Anderson, and Zelazo, 2011), and, therefore, the results may be robust. One possible interpretation is that the inferior prefrontal regions should be prepared during the preswitch phase for successful cognitive shifting during the postswitch phase. Activation during the preswitch phase, combined with the activation during the postswitch phase, may contribute to rule-switching in young children. The second interpretation is that the sustained activation may reflect deliberate selection processes of the task rules. In both phases, children may actively select 1 rule (e.g., shape) out of 2 rules (shape and color rules). With this idea, the inferior prefrontal activation may reflect the representations of the higher-order rules, which is consistent with cognitive explanations of the DCCS tasks by Zelazo and colleagues (Zelazo et al., 2003).

The second important set of results was that there might be individual differences in the development of prefrontal function during preschool ages. Children in the pass group activated the right prefrontal regions at Time 1 and then recruited bilateral inferior prefrontal regions at Time 2. Children in the perseverate group showed no significant activation in the prefrontal regions at Time 1 and recruited the left inferior prefrontal regions at Time 2 when they passed the DCCS tasks. It is likely that unilateral prefrontal activation was sufficient to perform the DCCS. However, it should be noted that 3-year-old children in the pass group (who performed the DCCS earlier) recruited the right inferior prefrontal areas. Children in the perseverate group who performed the task 1 year later than those in the pass group recruited the left prefrontal regions. These results suggested that right inferior prefrontal areas may be relatively dominant in cognitive-shifting tasks and left inferior prefrontal areas may support or compensate for right inferior prefrontal activations. In other words, children in the perseverate group failed to activate the right prefrontal regions for some reason, and, therefore, they could not pass the DCCS task at 3 years of age. However, they could activate the left prefrontal regions at 4 years of age, which resulted in successful performances on the DCCS task. The issue of laterality is again discussed in the final section.

TASK DEMAND AND PREFRONTAL ACTIVATION

Next, we examined whether the activation of inferior prefrontal regions may depend on the demands of cognitive shifting in young children (Moriguchi & Hiraki, in submission). We selected the advanced version of the DCCS (referred to as the ADCCS) to index the difficult version of the cognitive-shifting task (Zelazo, 2006). In the ADCCS, children need to switch flexibly between 2 incompatible rules within the same set. Half of the test cards have a border around them, while the other half does not (Figure 4). Children are asked to sort according to 1 rule if the card has a border and according to another rule if the card has no border. In these studies, children typically show more difficulty performing the ADCCS task than the standard DCCS task (Hongwanishkul, Happaney, Lee, and Zelazo, 2005).

Five-year-old children and adult participants were asked to perform the DCCS task and the ADCCS tasks, and neural activation during the tasks was examined with NIRS. In order to compare brain activation between the DCCS and ADCCS tasks, we averaged the data of the pre- and post-switch phases of the DCCS task and the data of all of the test phases of the ADCCS task. At the behavioral level, adult participants performed both tasks quite easily. However, 5-year-old children showed difficulty in performing the ADCCS compared to the DCCS, the performance of which was consistent with those of the previous studies (Hongwanishkul et al., 2005). At the neural level, adults showed significant changes in oxy-Hb levels in the right and left inferior prefrontal regions during the task phases compared to those during the control phases during both DCCS and ADCCS tasks. Direct comparisons of brain activations between the DCCS and ADCCS tasks revealed that the mean changes in oxy-Hb were significantly higher during the ADCCS task than during the DCCS task in the right and left inferior prefrontal regions (Figure 5A). For the children, the NIRS recordings revealed that the children showed significant changes in oxy-Hb levels in the right and left inferior prefrontal regions during the DCCS tasks and during the ADCCS task. A direct comparison of the brain activation patterns between the DCCS and ADCCS tasks revealed that the children engaged different brain regions depending on the task (Figure 5B). During the DCCS task, the children exhibited greater changes in oxy-Hb levels in the right prefrontal areas than during the ADCCS task. Conversely, in the left prefrontal areas, significant oxy-Hb increases were observed during the ADCCS task compared to during the DCCS task.

In this study, adults showed significantly stronger bilateral inferior prefrontal activation during the ADCCS task than during the DCCS task. This may have been due to the different demands on cognitive shifting across the tasks. In the DCCS task, the participants used a single rule (color rule or shape rule) during the test phases. Conversely, in the ADCCS task, the participants had to use 2 rules (a color rule and a shape rule) during 1 test phase. Therefore, the participants had to switch their mental sets more flexibly in the ADCCS task than in the standard DCCS task. In fact, the behavioral results showed that the participants took more time to complete the ADCCS task than the DCCS task.

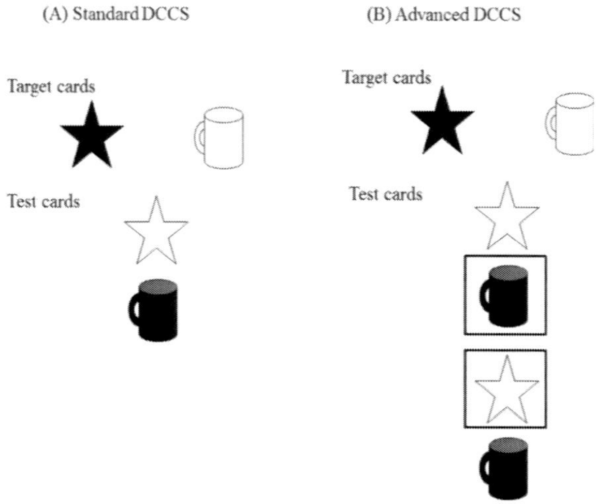

Figure 4. Stimuli used in *(A)* the Dimensional Change Card Sort (DCCS) task and *(B)* the advanced DCCS (ADCCS) task.

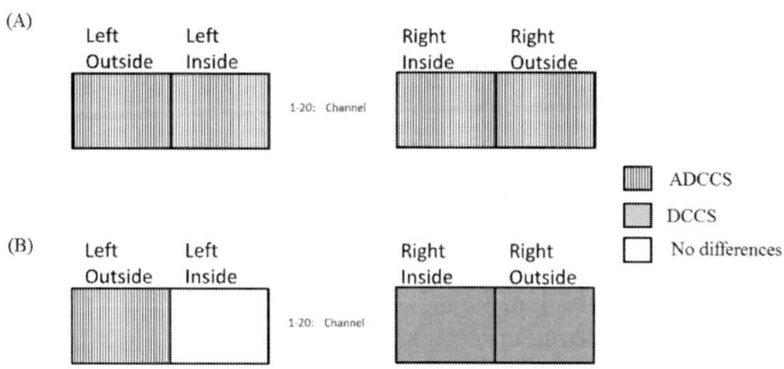

Figure 5. Differences in brain activation between the DCCS task and ADCCS task. *(A)* shows the brain activations in the adults, and *(B)* shows the brain activations in the 5-year-old children. The border areas highlight areas where stronger activations were observed during the ADCCS task than in the DCCS task. The gray areas highlight the areas where stronger activations were observed during the DCCS task than in the ADCCS task. The white areas highlight the areas where no significant differences were observed between the tasks.

In contrast, children showed significantly stronger right inferior prefrontal activation during the DCCS task, but they also exhibited stronger left inferior prefrontal activation during the ADCCS task. These laterality effects may be similar to those observed in the second study. Above, we suggested that the right inferior prefrontal regions might be dominant during the DCCS task while the left prefrontal regions may support or compensate for the right regions. Similar interpretations could be applied to the results of the present study. Five-year-old children activated the right inferior prefrontal regions in a standard cognitive shifting task (i.e., the DCCS). However, they may have needed an additional effort for the more difficult task and thus recruited the left inferior prefrontal regions in order to support the right prefrontal regions.

EF IN CHILDREN WITH AUTISM

Neuroimaging research with NIRS might also contribute to our understanding of developmental disorders, such as Autism spectrum disorder (ASD). ASD is characterized by deficits in social interaction and communication and restricted, repeated, and stereotyped interests and behaviors (American Psychiatric Association, 2000). There are several cognitive theories to explain the deficits of ASD, but 1 theory that might be related to the stereotyped behavior involves EF (Hill, 2004). Some previous studies have revealed that patients with ASD exhibit difficulty with cognitive shifting during the WCST (Ozonoff et al., 1994, but see also Nydén et al., 1999). These studies have suggested that children with ASD may have functional and anatomical deficits in the prefrontal cortex. However, there have been few brain imaging studies of young children with ASD. Thus, we aimed to examine whether there are behavioral and neural differences in cognitive shifting between typically developing (TD) children and ASD children with NIRS (Yasumura et al., 2012).

Seven- to 12-year-old ASD children and aged-matched TD children were asked to perform the ADCCS tasks, and the neural activity in the prefrontal cortex was examined with NIRS. Reading comprehension abilities that was assessed by the Kaufman Assessment Battery for Children (K-ABC) and nonverbal intelligence that was indexed by Raven's Colored Progressive Matrices (RCPM) test were also matched between the groups. The behavioral results revealed that ASD children performed the ADCCS significantly worse than TD children did. ASD children had significantly less correct answers, and they took significantly more time to perform the task compared to TD children. The NIRS results exhibited significant differences in the prefrontal activation between the groups. Consistent with our previous data, TD children exhibited significant bilateral prefrontal activation during the ADCCS. In contrast, ASD children showed significant left prefrontal activation, but the right prefrontal regions were not significantly activated. A direct comparison between the groups revealed significant differences between the groups in the right prefrontal regions. Finally, we examined whether the severity of ASD correlated to the behavioral and neural results. The severity of ASD was indexed by the Pervasive Developmental Disorders Autism Society Japan Rating Scale (PARS), which is a questionnaire on clinical conditions during both infancy and childhood (present). As a result, the scores during both infancy and the present significantly and negatively correlated with the behavioral and neural results. The number of correct answers in the ADCCS was negatively and significantly correlated with the scores on the PARS during both infancy and childhood. Moreover, activation in the right prefrontal areas significantly and negatively correlated with the scores on the PARS during infancy and childhood. That is, the severity of ASD was related to activation in the prefrontal areas and cognitive shifting. Taken together, these results showed that ASD children may have some difficulty with cognitive shifting at the behavioral and neural level.

CONCLUSION AND FURTHER DIRECTION

We reported the results of several experiments that examined the relationship between EF and prefrontal areas in young children and adult participants. As a result, both children and adult participants significantly activated the inferior prefrontal regions when they performed cognitive-shifting tasks, such as the DCCS. Importantly, younger TD children and ASD children who showed some difficulty with the tasks were less likely to activate the prefrontal regions. Taken together, our research suggests that activation in the prefrontal regions may be important for successful cognitive shifting in young children.

The next step is to determine how the development of prefrontal function may be related to other aspects of cognitive and social development. It has been shown that the development of EF correlates with the development of socio-cognitive skills, such as the theory of mind, communicative skills, and emotional regulation (Carlson and Moses, 2001; Dempster, 1992; Eisenberg et al., 1997; Moriguchi, Okanda, and Itakura, 2008). Given the correlational evidence, researchers have suggested that EF may contribute to the emergence of such skills (Moses, 2005). However, the exact mechanisms of such a relationship are still unclear. Our brain imaging technique may contribute to the understanding of such relationships. For example, it is possible that the prefrontal activations may help to activate the brain regions that are important for a given task.

There are several issues that should be addressed in future research. One important issue is laterality. In our study, children recruited left regions in more demanding tasks (the ADCCS) compared to easier tasks (the standard DCCS). In addition, ASD children recruited left prefrontal regions in the ADCCS. These results indicated that right prefrontal regions may be dominant for cognitive shifting in young children and left prefrontal regions may compensate for right prefrontal regions. The role of left inferior prefrontal regions should be discussed in terms of the development of inner speech. Inner speech refers to the activity of talking to oneself in silence, which contrasts to private speech (talking to oneself aloud). Both inner speech and private speech play an important role in self-regulative behaviors (Vygotsky, 1987). Indeed, children are likely to produce private speech during more demanding self-regulatory tasks (Kray, Eber, and Lindenberger, 2004; Luria, 1969). Moreover, there is evidence that verbalization may facilitate performances on EF tasks. For example, labeling the second rule in the DCCS task improved performances in the 3-year-olds (Kirkham et al., 2003). The performances of children in task switching has been shown to be significantly facilitated by verbal self-instructions (Kray, Eber, and Karbach, 2008). Importantly, a developmental shift from overt self-talk (private speech) to covert speech (inner speech) during early childhood has been shown (Manfra and Winsler, 2006). Thus, it is possible that children may produce inner speech when they are faced with difficult task-switching situations, such as in the ADCCS task, which may activate left inferior prefrontal regions. Indeed, adult participants recruit the left inferior frontal gyrus (Broca's area) when they produce inner speech (Baciu, Rubin, Décorps, and Segebarth, 1999; Hinke et al., 1993; Morin and Michaud, 2007). Thus, it is possible that activation in left prefrontal areas may reflect children's inner speech when switching from 1 rule to the other.

The second issue is that it is possible that other brain regions may be activated during these tasks. Given the limitation of our NIRS system, we focused on the role of the inferior prefrontal regions in the development of EF. However, Morton et al. (2009) reported with fMRI that school-aged children showed significant activation of the superior parietal cortex, dorsolateral prefrontal cortex, and presupplementary motor regions during the DCCS task. Furthermore, Monchi et al. (2001) have revealed that the dorsolateral prefrontal cortex and parietal cortex are significantly activated in adults during the WCST. Thus, we should examine activation in other brain regions in young children during cognitive-shifting tasks.

Third, developmental disorders other than ASD should be examined with our methodology. Attention-deficit hyperactivity disorder (ADHD) is a developmental disease that is characterized by inattention, hyperactivity, and impulsivity (American Psychiatric Association, 2000). There is ample behavioral evidence that children with ADHD show defects in EF (Barkley, 1997). Recently, it has been hypothesized that patients with ADHD may have functional deficits in the prefrontal cortex (Bush, Valera, and Seidman, 2005). However, it is still unclear when and how children with ADHD exhibit this deficit in prefrontal function. We are now addressing this issue with our NIRS technique. Further research is needed to examine the neural basis of executive function in children with developmental disorders, such as ASD and ADHD, and to apply the findings to clinical situations.

ACKNOWLEDGEMENT

The Figure 2 and 3 were reprented from *Developmental Cognitive Neuroscience*, 1, Moriguchi, Y., & Hiraki, K. (2011), Longitudinal development of prefrontal function during early childhood, 153-162, Copyright (2011), with permission from Elsevier.

REFERENCES

American Psychiatric Association. (2000). *Diagnostic and Statistical Manual of Mental Disorders* (4th ed., text rev.). Washington DC: American Psychiatric Association.

Baciu, M. V., Rubin, C., Décorps, M. A., and Segebarth, C. M. (1999). fMRI assessment of hemispheric language dominance using a simple inner speech paradigm. *NMR in Biomedicine, 12*(5), 293-298. doi: 10.1002/(sici)1099-1492(199908)12:5<293::aid-nbm573>3.0.co;2-6.

Barkley, R. A. (1997). Behavioral inhibition, sustained attention, and executive functions: Constructing a unifying theory of ADHD. *Psychological Bulletin, 121*(1), 65-94.

Bush, G., Valera, E. M., and Seidman, L. J. (2005). Functional neuroimaging of attention-deficit/hyperactivity disorder: a review and suggested future directions. *Biological Psychiatry, 57*(11), 1273-1284.

Carlson, S. M. (2005). Developmentally sensitive measures of executive function in preschool children. *Developmental Neuropsychology, 28*(2), 595-616.

Carlson, S. M., and Moses, L. J. (2001). Individual differences in inhibitory control and children's theory of mind. *Child Development, 72*(4), 1032-1053.

Crone, E. A., Donohue, S. E., Honomichl, R., Wendelken, C., and Bunge, S. A. (2006). Brain Regions Mediating Flexible Rule Use during

Development. *Journal of Neuroscience, 26*(43), 11239-11247. doi: 10.1523/jneurosci.2165-06.2006.

Dempster, F. N. (1992). The Rise and Fall of the Inhibitory Mechanism: Toward a Unified Theory of Cognitive-Development and Aging. *Developmental Review, 12*(1), 45-75.

Diamond, A. (2002). Normal development of prefrontal cortex from birth to young adulthood: Cognitive functions, anatomy, and biochemistry. In D. T. Stuss and R. T. Knight (Eds.), *Principles of frontal lobe function* (pp. 466-503). New York: Oxford University Press.

Diamond, A., and Taylor, C. (1996). Development of an aspect of executive control: Development of the abilities to remember what I said and to "Do as I say, not as I do". *Developmental Psychobiology, 29*(4), 315-334.

Eisenberg, N., Guthrie, I. K., Fabes, R. A., Reiser, M., Murphy, B. C., Holgren, R., ... Losoya, S. (1997). The relations of regulation and emotionality to resiliency and competent social functioning in elementary school children. *Child Development, 68*(2), 295-311.

Espinet, S. D., Anderson, J. E., and Zelazo, P. D. (2012). N2 amplitude as a neural marker of executive function in young children: an ERP study of children who switch versus perseverate on the Dimensional Change Card Sort. *Developmental Cognitive Neuroscience 2*(Suppl. 1): S49-S58.

Garon, N., Bryson, S. E., and Smith, I. M. (2008). Executive function in preschoolers: A review using an integrative framework. *Psychological Bulletin, 134*(1), 31-60. doi: 10.1037/0033-2909.134.1.31.

Gerstadt, C. L., Hong, Y. J., and Diamond, A. (1994). The Relationship between Cognition and Action: Performance of Children 3 1/2-7 Years Old on a Stroop-Like Day-Night Test. *Cognition, 53*(2), 129-153.

Giedd, J. N., Blumenthal, J., Jeffries, N. O., Castellanos, F. X., Liu, H., Zijdenbos, A., ... Rapoport, J. L. (1999). Brain development during childhood and adolescence: a longitudinal MRI study. *Nature Neuroscience, 2*(10), 861-863. doi: 10.1038/13158.

Gogtay, N., Giedd, J. N., Lusk, L., Hayashi, K. M., Greenstein, D., Vaituzis, A. C., ... Thompson, P. M. (2004). Dynamic mapping of human cortical development during childhood through early adulthood. *Proceedings of the National Academy of Sciences of the United States of America, 101*(21), 8174-8179.

Hill, E. L. (2004). Executive dysfunction in autism. *Trends in Cognitive Sciences, 8*(1), 26-32. doi: 10.1016/j.tics.2003.11.003.

Hinke, R. M., Hu, X., Stillman, A. E., Kim, S. G., Merkle, H., Salmi, R., and Ugurbil, K. (1993). Functional magnetic resonance imaging of Broca's area during internal speech. *Neuroreport, 4*(6), 675-678.

Hongwanishkul, D., Happaney, K. R., Lee, W. S., and Zelazo, P. D. (2005). Assessment of hot and cool executive function in young children: Age-related changes and individual differences. *Developmental Neuropsychology, 28*(2), 617-644.

Huizinga, M., Dolan, C. V., and van der Molen, M. W. (2006). Age-related change in executive function: Developmental trends and a latent variable analysis. *Neuropsychologia, 44*(11), 2017-2036. doi: 10.1016/ j.neuropsychologia.2006.01.010.

Kirkham, N. Z., Cruess, L., and Diamond, A. (2003). Helping children apply their knowledge to their behavior on a dimension-switching task. *Developmental Science, 6*(5), 449-467.

Konishi, S., Nakajima, K., Uchida, I., Kameyama, M., Nakahara, K., Sekihara, K., and Miyashita, Y. (1998). Transient activation of inferior prefrontal cortex during cognitive set shifting. *Nature Neuroscience, 1*(1), 80-84.

Kray, J., Eber, J., and Karbach, J. (2008). Verbal self-instructions in task switching: a compensatory tool for action-control deficits in childhood and old age? *Developmental Science, 11*(2), 223-236.

Kray, J., Eber, J., and Lindenberger, U. (2004). Age differences in executive functioning across the lifespan: The role of verbalization in task preparation. *Acta Psychologica, 115*(2-3), 143-165. doi: 10.1016/j.actpsy.2003.12.001.

Lehto, J. E., Juujarvi, P., Kooistra, L., and Pulkkinen, L. (2003). Dimensions of executive functioning: Evidence from children. *British Journal of Developmental Psychology, 21*(1), 59-80.

Luria, A. R. (1969). Speech development and the formation of mental processes. In M. Cole and I. Maltzman (Eds.), *A handbook of contemporary Soviet psychology*. New York: Basic Books.

Manfra, L., and Winsler, A. (2006). Preschool children's awareness of private speech. *International Journal of Behavioral Development, 30*(6), 537-549. doi: 10.1177/ 0165025406072902.

Matsuda, G., and Hiraki, K. (2006). Sustained decrease in oxygenated hemoglobin during video games in the dorsal prefrontal cortex: A NIRS study of children. *NeuroImage, 29*(3), 706-711.

Miyake, A., and Friedman, N. P. (2012). The Nature and Organization of Individual Differences in Executive Functions: Four General Conclusions. *Current Directions in Psychological Science, 21*(1), 8-14. doi: 10.1177/0963721411429458.

Miyake, A., Friedman, N. P., Emerson, M. J., Witzki, A. H., Howerter, A., and Wager, T. D. (2000). The unity and diversity of executive functions and their contributions to complex "frontal lobe" tasks: A latent variable analysis. *Cognitive Psychology, 41*(1), 49-100. doi: 10.1006/cogp.1999.0734.

Monchi, O., Petrides, M., Petre, V., Worsley, K., and Dagher, A. (2001). Wisconsin card sorting revisited: Distinct neural circuits participating in different stages of the task identified by event-related functional magnetic resonance imaging. *Journal of Neuroscience, 21*(19), 7733-7741.

Moriguchi, Y. (2012). The effect of social observation on children's inhibitory control. *Journal of Experimental Child Psychology, 113*(2), 248-258. doi: http://dx.doi.org/ 10.1016/j.jecp.2012.06.002.

Moriguchi, Y., and Hiraki, K. (2009). Neural origin of cognitive shifting in young children. *Proceedings of the National Academy of Sciences of the United States of America, 106*(14), 6017-6021.

Moriguchi, Y., and Hiraki, K. (2011). Longitudinal development of prefrontal function during early childhood. *Developmental Cognitive Neuroscience, 1*(2), 153-162.

Moriguchi, Y., Lee, K., and Itakura, S. (2007). Social transmission of disinhibition in young children. *Developmental Science, 10*(4), 481-491. doi: 10.1111/j.1467-7687.2007. 00601.x.

Moriguchi, Y., Okanda, M., and Itakura, S. (2008). Young children's yes bias: How does it relate to verbal ability, inhibitory control, and theory of mind? *First Language, 28*(4), 431-442. doi: 10.1177/0142723708092413.

Morin, A., and Michaud, J. (2007). Self-awareness and the left inferior frontal gyrus: Inner speech use during self-related processing. *Brain Research Bulletin, 74*(6), 387-396. doi: DOI: 10.1016/j.brainresbull.2007.06.013.

Morton, J. B., Bosma, R., and Ansari, D. (2009). Age-related changes in brain activation associated with dimensional shifts of attention: An fMRI study. *NeuroImage, 46*(1), 249-256.

Moses, L. J. (2005). Executive Functioning and Children's Theories of Mind. In B. F. Malle and S. D. Hodges (Eds.), *Other minds: How humans bridge the divide between self and others.* (pp. 11-25). New York, NY: Guilford Press.

Nydén, A., Gillberg, C., Hjelmquist, E., and Heiman, M. (1999). Executive function/attention deficits in boys with Asperger syndrome, attention disorder and reading/writing disorder. *Autism, 3*(3), 213-228.

Oh, S., and Lewis, C. (2008). Korean preschoolers' advanced inhibitory control and its relation to other executive skills and mental state understanding. *Child Development, 79*(1), 80-99.

Okamoto, M., Dan, H., Sakamoto, K., Takeo, K., Shimizu, K., Kohno, S., ... Dan, I. (2004). Three-dimensional probabilistic anatomical cranio-cerebral correlation via the international 10-20 system oriented for transcranial functional brain mapping. *NeuroImage, 21*(1), 99-111.

Ozonoff, S., Strayer, D. L., McMahon, W. M., and Filloux, F. (1994). Executive Function Abilities in Autism and Tourette Syndrome: An Information Processing Approach. *Journal of Child Psychology and Psychiatry, 35*(6), 1015-1032. doi: 10.1111/j.1469-7610.1994.tb01807.x.

Rueda, M. R., Rothbart, M. K., McCandliss, B. D., Saccomanno, L., and Posner, M. I. (2005). Training, maturation, and genetic influences on the development of executive attention. *Proceedings of the National Academy of Sciences of the United States of America, 102*(41), 14931-14936. doi: 10.1073/pnas.0506897102.

Simpson, A., and Riggs, K. J. (2005). Factors responsible for performance on the day-night task: response set or semantics? *Developmental Science, 8*(4), 360-371.

Simpson, A., and Riggs, K. J. (2007). Under what conditions do young children have difficulty inhibiting manual actions? *Developmental Psychology, 43*(2), 417-428. doi: 10.1037/0012-1649.43.2.417.

Strangman, G., Culver, J. P., Thompson, J. H., and Boas, D. A. (2002). A Quantitative Comparison of Simultaneous BOLD fMRI and NIRS Recordings during Functional Brain Activation. *NeuroImage, 17*(2), 719-731.

Tsujimoto, S. (2008). The prefrontal cortex: Functional neural development during early childhood. *Neuroscientist, 14*(4), 345-358.

Vygotsky, L. S. (1987). Thinking and speech. In R. W. Rieber and A. S. Carton (Eds.), *The collected works of L.S. Vygotsky, Volume 1: Problems of general psychology* (pp. 39-285). New York: Plenum Press.

Wiebe, S. A., Espy, K. A., and Charak, D. (2008). Using confirmatory factor analysis to understand executive control in preschool children: I. Latent structure. *Developmental Psychology, 44*(2), 575-587. doi: 10.1037/0012-1649.44.2.575.

Yasumura, A., Kokubo, N., Yamamoto, H., Yasumura, Y., Moriguchi, Y., Nakagawa, E., ... Hiraki, K. (2012). Neurobehavioral and hemodynamic evaluation of cognitive shifting in children with autism spectrum disorder. *Journal of Behavioral and Brain Science, 2*(4), 463-470.

Zelazo, P. D. (2006). The Dimensional Change Card Sort (DCCS): a method of assessing executive function in children. *Nature Protocols, 1*(1), 297-301.

Zelazo, P. D., Frye, D., and Rapus, T. (1996). An age-related dissociation between knowing rules and using them. *Cognitive Development, 11*(1), 37-63.

Zelazo, P. D., Muller, U., Frye, D., Marcovitch, S., Argitis, G., Boseovski, J., …Sutherland, A. (2003). The development of executive function in early childhood. *Monographs of the Society for Research in Child Development, 68*(3), vii-137.

INDEX

A

D

E

J

K

L

N

O

P

Q

R

S

T